Cafer's Mood Stabilizers and Antiepileptic Drugs:

Drug interactions and trade/generic name pairings of medications for bipolar and seizure disorders

First Edition, 2020

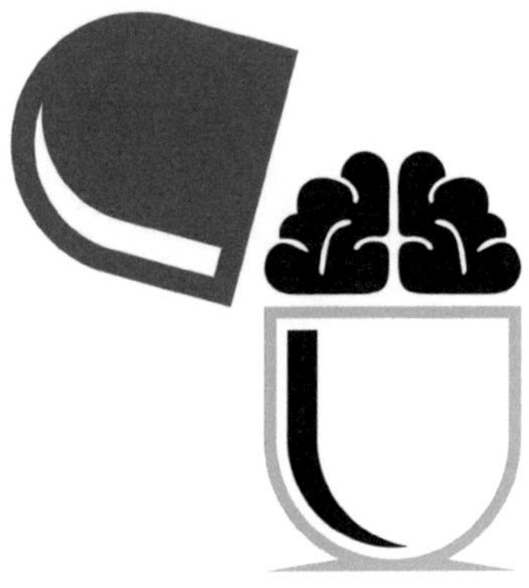

Author: Jason Cafer, MD

Editor: Julianna Link, PA-C

Cafer's Mood Stabilizers and Antiepileptics:
Drug Interactions and Trade/generic Name Pairings of Medications for Bipolar and Seizure Disorders (Visualize to Memorize series)

First Edition

Author: Jason Cafer, MD

Editor: Julianna Link, PA-C

Illustrations: Coccus from 99Designs

Cover design: BengsWorks from 99Designs

Licensed images: Shutterstock and Wikimedia Commons

ISBN: 978-1-7350901-0-8

Contact: jason@cafermed.com

This book includes a subset of 46 medication mascots from *Cafer's Psychopharmacology*, which contains 270. Medications chosen for this edition include lithium, FDA-approved medications for seizure disorders, and all available benzodiazepines and barbiturates.

Contents of this book

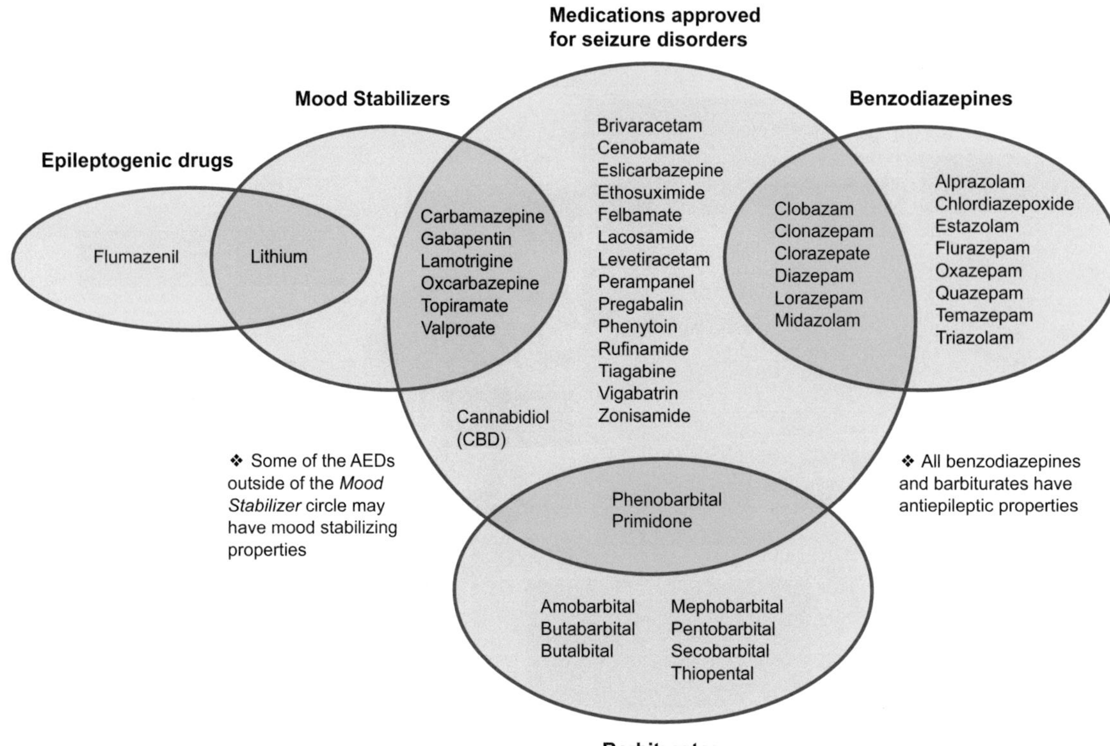

The scope of drug interaction information is limited to what can be digested and applied to routine clinical practice. There are countless unmentioned drug-drug interactions that could be relevant for some patients but are omitted because the amount of material would be overwhelming.

This book is focused on medications, not overarching psychiatric care. Although chemicals are necessary for treatment of mania or acute psychosis, pharmacologic treatment of depression/anxiety/insomnia/etc is not always the best medicine. Always consider interventions including cognitive behavioral therapy, diet, exercise, mindfulness, sleep hygiene, etc. For bipolar mania, Virtual Darkness Therapy is an experimental non-pharmacological treatment described on page 48.

Dosing recommendations are for healthy adults, and <u>may differ from FDA prescribing guidelines</u>. Refer to other sources for treatment of children, older adults, pregnancy/breastfeeding and renal/hepatic insufficiency.

Every effort has been made to provide accurate and up-to-date information. Author/editors/publisher/reviewers disclaim all liability for direct or consequential damages resulting from the use of this material. Readers are encouraged to confirm information with other sources before incorporating it into your prescribing practice. Information should be compared with official instructions from the drug manufacturer.

Complete contents of *Cafer's Psychopharmacology*. The content included in this edition is highlighted.

Chapter 1
Interactions 5
P-glycoprotein 9
CYP1A2 10
CYP2B6 12
CYP2C9 13
CYP2C19 14
CYP2D6 15
CYP3A4 16
UGT interactions (lamotrigine) 17
Meds with minimal interactions 18
Interaction table 20
Symbols defined 22

Chapter 2
Stabilizers / Antiepileptics 23
Mood stabilizers 23
Lithium 24
Antiepileptic drugs (AEDs) 27
Lamotrigine (Lamictal) 28
Valproate (Depakene, Depakote) 29
Carbamazepine (Tegretol) 31
Oxcarbazepine (Trileptal) 33
Gabapentin (Neurontin) 34
Pregabalin (Lyrica) 35
Topiramate (Topamax) 36
Levetiracetam (Keppra) 37
Phenytoin (Dilantin) 38
Zonisamide (Zonegran) 39
Lacosamide (Vimpat) 40
Ethosuximide (Zarontin) 40
Eslicarbazepine (Aptiom) 41
Rufinamide (Banzel) 41
Felbamate (Felbatol) 42
Brivaracetam (Briviact) 42
Tiagabine (Gabitril) 43
Perampanel (Fycompa) 43
Cenobamate (Xcopri) 44
Vigabatrin (Sabril) 45
Cannabidiol (CBD, Epidiolex) 46
Epileptogenic drugs 47
Virtual darkness therapy 48

Chapter 3
Barbiturates 49
Phenobarbital (Luminal) 50
Primidone (Mysoline) 50
Butabarbital (Butisol) 51
Mephobarbital (Mebaral) 51
Butalbital combo (Fioricet) 52
Secobarbital (Seconal) 52
Pentobarbital (Nembutal) 52
Amobarbital (Amytal) 53
Thiopental (Sodium Pentothal) 53

Chapter 4
Benzodiazepines 55
Alprazolam (Xanax) 57
Clonazepam (Klonopin) 58
Lorazepam (Ativan) 58
Diazepam (Valium) 59
Temazepam (Restoril) 59
Chlordiazepoxide (Librium) 60
Triazolam (Halcion) 60
Clorazepate (Tranxene) 61
Oxazepam (Serax) 61
Flurazepam (Dalmane) 62
Estazolam (Prosom) 62
Quazepam (Doral) 63
Clobazam (Onfi) 63
Midazolam (Versed) 64
Flumazenil (Romazicon) 64

Chapter 5
Anxiolytics / Hypnotics 65
Buspirone (Buspar) 66
Z-drugs 67
DEA-controlled substances 67
Zolpidem (Ambien) 68
Eszopiclone (Lunesta) 69
Zaleplon (Sonata) 69
Melatonin 70
Ramelteon (Rozerem) 71
Tasimelteon (Hetlioz) 71
Orexin (hypocretin) 72
Narcolepsy 72
Suvorexant (Belsomra) 73
Lemborexant (Dayvigo) 74
Sodium Oxybate (Xyrem, GHB) 75
Propofol (Diprivan) 76

Chapter 6
Intro to antidepressants 77
Toxicity of antidepressant overdose 80
Sexual side effects 80
Serotonin syndrome 81, 128
QT prolongation 82

Chapter 7
Tricyclics (TCAs) 83
Amitriptyline (Elavil) 84
Nortriptyline (Pamelor) 85
Doxepin (Sinequan, Silenor) 86
Imipramine (Tofranil) 87
Clomipramine (Anafranil) 88
Desipramine (Norpramin) 89
Protriptyline (Vivactil) 89
Amoxapine (Asendin) 90
Maprotiline (Ludiomil) 91
Trimipramine (Surmontil) 91

Chapter 8
Modern Antidepressants 93
Sertraline (Zoloft) 94
Escitalopram (Lexapro) 95
Citalopram (Celexa) 96
Fluoxetine (Prozac) 97
Paroxetine (Paxil) 98
Fluvoxamine (Luvox) 99
SNRIs / atypical antidepressants 100
Duloxetine (Cymbalta) 101
Venlafaxine (Effexor) 102
Desvenlafaxine (Pristiq, Khedezla) 103
Milnacipran (Savella) 104
Levomilnacipran (Fetzima) 105
Trazodone (Desyrel, Oleptro) 106
Nefazodone (Serzone) 107
Mirtazapine (Remeron) 108
California Rocket Fuel 109
Vortioxetine (Trintellix) 110
Vilazodone (Viibryd) 111
Serotonin discontinuation syndrome 112
NRIs, NDRIs, DNRIs 113
Atomoxetine (Strattera) 114
Bupropion (Wellbutrin) 115

Chapter 9
MAOIs 117
Isocarboxazid (Marplan) 118
Phenelzine (Nardil) 119
Tranylcypromine (Parnate) 119
Selegiline transdermal (EMSAM) 120

Chapter 10
Others (depression) 121
L-methylfolate (Deplin) 121
Ketamine (Ketalar) 122
Esketamine (Spravato) 123
Brexanolone (Zulresso) 124
St John's Wort (SJW) 125

Chapter 11
Intro to antipsychotics 127
Neuroleptic malignant syndrome 128
1st and 2nd generation antipsychotics ... 130

Chapter 12
1st Gen Antipsychotics 131
Haloperidol (Haldol) 132
Chlorpromazine (Thorazine) 133
Perphenazine (Trilafon) 134
Fluphenazine (Prolixin) 136
Thiothixene (Navane) 137
Loxapine (Loxitane) 137
Trifluoperazine (Stelazine) 138
Thioridazine (Mellaril) 139
Pimozide (Orap) 140
Molindone (Moban) 140
Antiemetics that block D2 receptors 141
Prochlorperazine (Compazine) 141
Promethazine (Phenergan) 142
Metoclopramide (Reglan) 143
Trimethobenzamide (Tigan) 143

Chapter 13
2nd Gen Antipsychotics 145
Quetiapine (Seroquel) 146
Aripiprazole (Abilify, Maintena, Aristada) 147
Risperidone (Risperdal, Consta) 148
Olanzapine (Zyprexa) 149
Lurasidone (Latuda) 150
Ziprasidone (Geodon) 151
Clozapine (Clozaril) 152
Brexpiprazole (Rexulti) 153
Cariprazine (Vraylar) 154
Paliperidone (Invega, Sustenna)......... 155
Iloperidone (Fanapt) 156
Asenapine (Saphris, Secuado) 157
Lumateperone (Caplyta) 158
Pimavanserin (Nuplazid) 159
Long-acting injectables 160

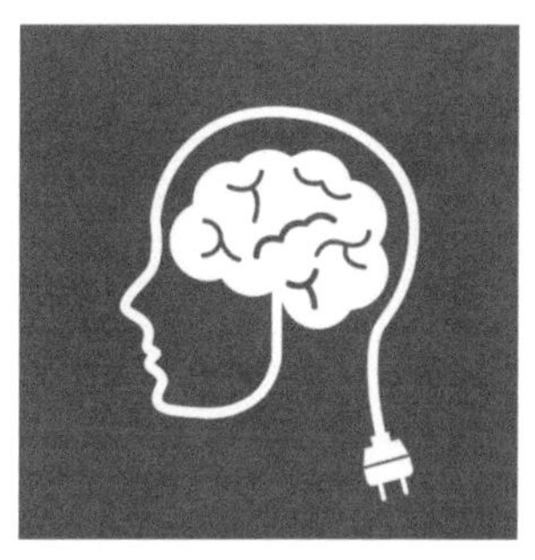

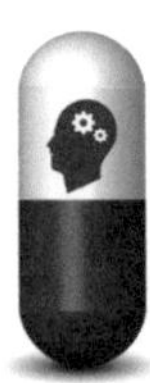

Chapter 14
Anticholinergics 161

Anticholinergic burden scale 162
Antihistamines 163
Diphenhydramine (Benadryl) 164
Doxylamine (Unisom) 164
Hydroxyzine (Vistaril, Atarax) 165
Meclizine (Antivert) 166
Dimenhydrinate (Dramamine) 166
Cyproheptadine (Periactin) 167
Anticholinergics 168
Benztropine (Cogentin) 169
Dicyclomine (Bentyl) 171
Hyoscyamine (Anaspaz, Levsin) 171
Scopolamine (Transderm Scōp) 171
Glycopyrrolate (Robinul) 172
Glycopyrronium (Qbrexza) 172
Oxybutynin (Ditropan) 173
Tolterodine (Detrol) 173
Solifenacin (Vesicare) 174
Fesoterodine (Toviaz) 174
Darifenacin (Enablex) 175
Trospium (Sanctura) 175
Atropine (Atropen, Atropisol) 176
Pupils – mydriasis and miosis 176

Chapter 15
Cognitive enhancers 177

Cognitive enhancers 177
Cholinergics 177
Donepezil (Aricept) 178
Rivastigmine (Exelon) 179
Galantamine (Razadyne) 179
Bethanechol (Urecholine) 180
Pilocarpine (Salagen) 181
Memantine (Namenda) 182
Namzaric (memantine + donepezil) 182

Chapter 16
Antihypertensives 183

Clonidine (Catapres, Kapvay) 183
Guanfacine (Tenex, Intuniv) 184
Lofexidine (Lucemyra) 185
Dexmedetomidine (Precedex) 185
Prazosin (Minipress) 186
Propranolol (Inderal) 187
Amlodipine (Norvasc) 188
Nimodipine (Nimotop) 188

Chapter 17
Muscle relaxants 189

Cyclobenzaprine (Flexeril) 190
Baclofen (Lioresal) 191
Methocarbamol (Robaxin) 192
Tizanidine (Zanaflex) 192
Metaxalone (Skelaxin) 193
Orphenadrine (Norflex) 193
Meprobamate (Miltown) 194
Carisoprodol (Soma) 195
Methaqualone (Quāālude) 196

Chapter 18
DA depleting agents 197

Tardive dyskinesia treatment 197
VMAT inhibitors 198
Tetrabenazine (Xenazine) 199
Deutetrabenazine (Austedo) 200
Valbenazine (Ingrezza) 200
Reserpine (Serpasil) 201

Chapter 19
Parkinson's disease 203

Carbidopa – levodopa (Sinemet) 206
Ropinirole (Requip) 207
Pramipexole (Mirapex) 208
Apomorphine (Apokyn) 209
Rotigotine (Neupro) 209
Bromocriptine (Parlodel) 210
Cabergoline (Dostinex) 210
Entacapone (Comtan) 211
Tolcapone (Tasmar) 211
Selegiline PO (Eldepryl) 212
Rasagiline (Azilect) 213
Safinamide (Xadago) 213
Amantadine (Symmetrel) 214
Istradefylline (Nourianz) 215

Chapter 20
Stimulants 217

Treatment of ADHD 218
Methylphenidate (Ritalin) 220
Dexmethylphenidate (Focalin) 221
Concerta 221
Aptensio XR 222
Jornay PM 222
Adhansia XR 223
Cotempla XR-ODT 223
Daytrana 224
Amphetamine salts (Adderall) 225
Dextroamphetamine (Dexedrine) 226
Adzenys XR-ODT 226
Lisdexamfetamine (Vyvanse) 227
Mydayis 227
Evekeo 228
Methamphetamine (Desoxyn) 228
Modafinil (Provigil) 229
Armodafinil (Nuvigil) 230
Solriamfetol (Sunosi) 230
Phentermine (Adipex) 231
Qsymia (phentermine + topiramate) 231
Lorcaserin (Belviq) 232
Pitolisant (Wakix) 233
Caffeine 234

Chapter 21
Addiction medicine 235

Nicotine 236
Varenicline (Chantix) 237
Dronabinol (THC, Marinol) 238
Disulfiram (Antabuse) 239
Acamprosate (Campral) 240
Dextromethorphan (DXM) 241
Nuedexta (DXM + quinidine) 242
Hallucinogens 243
LSD 244

Chapter 22
Opioids 245

Constipation treatment 246
Morphine (MS Contin) 247
Hydromorphone (Dilaudid) 247
Oxymorphone (Numorphan) 248
Hydrocodone/APAP (Vicodin) 248
Oxycodone/APAP (Percocet) 249
Codeine/APA (Tylenol #2,3,4) 250
Heroin (diamorphine) 251
Meperidine (Demerol) 252
Fentanyl (Duragesic) 252
Methadone (Dolophine) 253
Tramadol (Ultram) 254
Tapentadol (Nucynta) 255
Levorphanol (Levo-Dromoran) 256
Naltrexone (ReVia) 257
Naltrexone LAI (Vivitrol) 258
Low dose naltrexone 258
Contrave (naltrexone + bupropion) .. 259
Naloxone (Narcan) 260
Buprenorphine (Subutex, Suboxone) 261
Butorphanol (Stadol) 264
Pentazocine (Talwin) 264
Nalbuphine (Nubain) 265
Loperamide (Imodium) 266
Diphenoxylate/Atropine (Lomotil) 266

Chapter 23
Sexual dysfunction 267

Flibanserin (Addyi) 267
Bremelanotide (Vyleesi) 268
Sildenafil (Viagra) 269
Tadalafil (Cialis) 270
Vardenafil (Levitra) 270
Avanafil (Stendra) 270

Chapter 24
Antimicrobials 271

Fluconazole (Diflucan) 271
Minocycline (Minocin) 272
Clarithromycin (Biaxin).................... 272
Fluoroquinolones 273
Rifampin (Rifadin) 273

Chapter 25
Hormones 275

Levothyroxine (Synthroid, T4) 276
Liothyronine (Cytomel, T3) 277
Armour Thyroid 277
Oxytocin (Pitocin) 278
Tamoxifen (Nolvadex) 279
Raloxifene (Evista) 280

Chapter 26
Leftovers 281

Metformin (Glucophage) 281
Acetylcysteine (NAC) 282
Ondansetron (Zofran) 283
Sumatriptan (Imitrex) 284
Rizatriptan (Maxalt) 284
Fremanezumab (Ajovy) 285
Galcanezumab (Emgality)................ 285
Erenumab (Aimovig) 285
Omeprazole (Prilosec) 286

PHARMACODYNAMICS VS PHARMACOKINETICS

Drug-drug interactions fall into two main categories: **pharmacokinetic** and **pharmacodynamic**.

Pharmacodynamics is what a drug does to the body. Pharmacodynamic interactions are based on the drugs' mechanisms of action and do not involve alteration in blood levels of either interacting drug.

Pharmacokinetics is what the body does to a drug. Kinetic derives from the Greek verb *kinein*, "to move". In this case we're talking movement into and out of the body, for instance absorbing the chemical from the gut and processing it for excretion in urine or feces. Pharmacokinetic (PK) interactions are generally manifested by alteration of blood levels of one of the interacting drugs.

For simplicity's sake, let's drop the *pharmaco-* prefix and refer to these concepts as **kinetic** interactions and **dynamic** interactions.

PHARMACODYNAMIC INTERACTIONS

Dynamic interactions are intuitive if you understand how the interacting drugs work. Although dynamic interactions are understandable without silly pictures, here are a couple anyhow.

Dynamic interactions can be **additive/synergistic**, with enhanced effects brought about by combining medications with similar or complementary effects.

Like-minded "**dyn**os" ganging up to reduce blood pressure, which is an additive/synergistic effect.

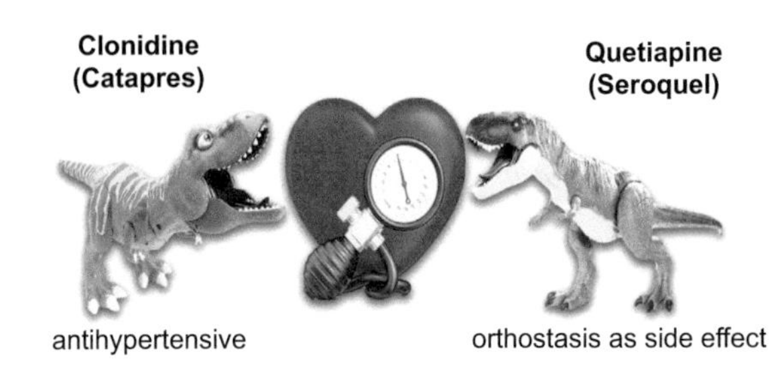

Other dynamic interactions are **antagonistic**, for instance combining a dopaminergic such as pramipexole (for restless legs) with an antidopaminergic like haloperidol (antipsychotic). Here's another example:

Fighting "**dyn**os" involved in an antagonistic interaction.

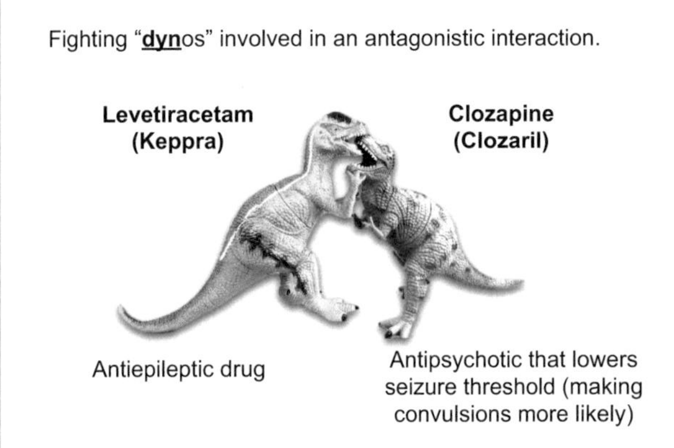

PHARMACOKINETIC INTERACTIONS

Kinetics involves the rate at which a drug gets into or out of the body or brain.

Drug-drug Interactions involving absorption are generally straightforward. For instance, anticholinergics slow gut motility and delay gastrointestinal absorption of other medications.

Kinetic interactions involving rate of elimination from the body are challenging to learn and daunting to memorize. It is important to consider these interactions to avoid underdosing or overdosing certain medications. This book tackles these tricky elimination interactions by illustrating:

❖ Phase I metabolism involving the six most important cytochrome P450 (CYP450) enzymes

❖ Phase II metabolism involving UGT enzymes, as applicable to lamotrigine (Lamictal)

❖ Renal clearance of lithium (page 26)

A mysterious type of kinetic interaction involves drugs getting across the blood-brain barrier, as is necessary for a psychiatric medication to take effect. If such an interaction is occurring, the effect will not be detectable in serum drug levels. This will be discussed in the context of P-glycoprotein (page 9).

CYTOCHROME P450 ENZYMES

In the liver, kinetic interactions predominantly involve **CYtochrome P450 enzymes**, **CYP** enzymes for short, which can be pronounced "sip". Instead of concerning yourself with the origin of P450 nomenclature, take a moment to contemplate this picture of Ken (kinetic) taking a "sip" (CYP).

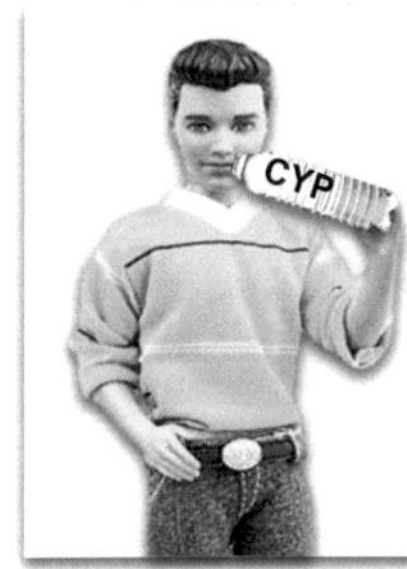

"Sip" (CYP) enzyme interactions are (pharmaco) "Ken-etic"

CYP enzymes, which reside primarily in the liver, make chemicals less lipid-soluble so they can be more easily excreted in urine or bile. Of over 50 CYP enzymes, six play a major role in the biotransformation of medications: 1A2, 2B6, 2C9, 2C19, 2D6 and 3A4. Our visual mnemonics will be built on the following phraseology:

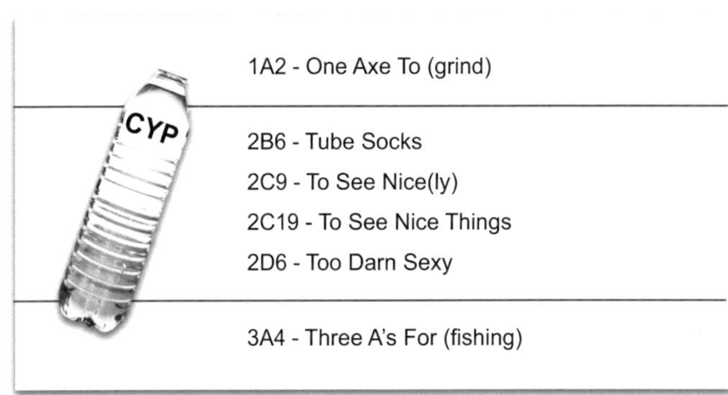

The three most important CYPs are **1A2, 2D6** and **3A4**. For psychiatrists, 2C19 can be important, while 2B6 and 2C9 are rarely significant.

SUBSTRATES

A drug that is biotransformed by a particular enzyme is referred to as a **substrate** of that enzyme. When the substrate is biotransformed (metabolized) it is then referred to as a **metabolite**.

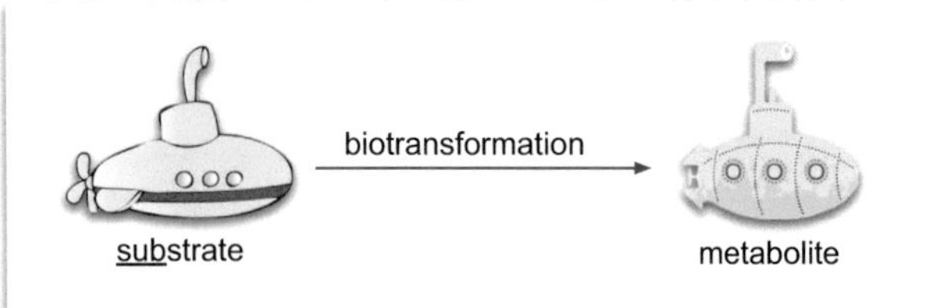

Each CYP enzyme can metabolize several substrates and most substrates can be metabolized by several CYP enzymes. Substrates are the "victims" of the interactions described in this chapter. Throughout this book we use the following visuals for CYP substrates:

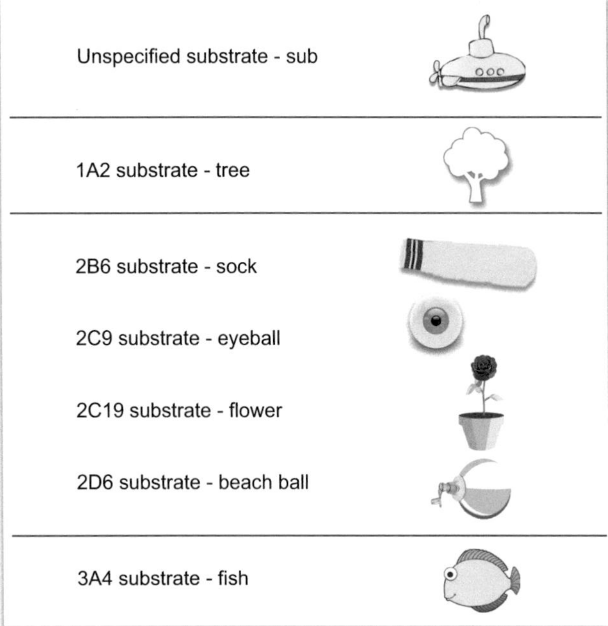

"Aggressor" medications affect how long victim substrates linger in the blood, and the relative serum concentration of parent drug (substrate) to metabolite. For a given enzyme, interfering medications (aggressors) are either in**D**ucers or in**H**ibitors. **InDucers** stimulate (in**D**uce) production of metabolic enzymes. **InHibitors** interfere with an enzyme's ability to metabolize other medications.

ENZYME INHIBITION

InHibition of an enzyme occurs when one drug (the in**H**ibitor) binds more tightly to the enzyme than the victim substrate binds. The in**H**ibitor itself may be metabolized by the enzyme, or act as a non-competitive inhibitor. When an inhibitor is bound to an enzyme, the victim substrate must find another enzyme to metabolize it, or hope that it can eventually be excreted unchanged. Strong inhibitors may cause the victim substrate to linger longer, prolonging the victim's half-life and elevating its concentration in the blood. For victim substrates that cross the blood brain barrier (as is necessary to be psychoactive), inhibition leads to increased drug concentration in the central nervous system.

Why is **H** being emphasized? Well, when an in**H**ibitor is added to an individual's medication regimen, levels of victim drugs can escalate (**H** for **H**igh). In**H**ibition takes effect quickly, within **H**ours (**H** for **H**urried), although the effect may not be clinically evident for 2 to 4 days, until the victim substrate accumulates.

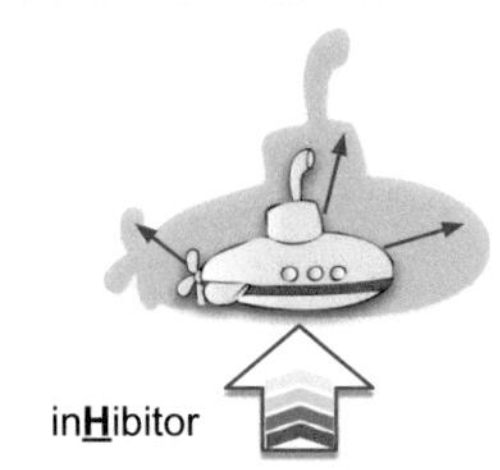

Increased concentration of substrate (and increased ratio of serum substrate:metabolite)

H for **H**igh and **H**urried, within 2- 4 hours, although the effect may not be clinically evident for 2 - 4 days

In**H**ibitors of CYP enzymes will be represented by:

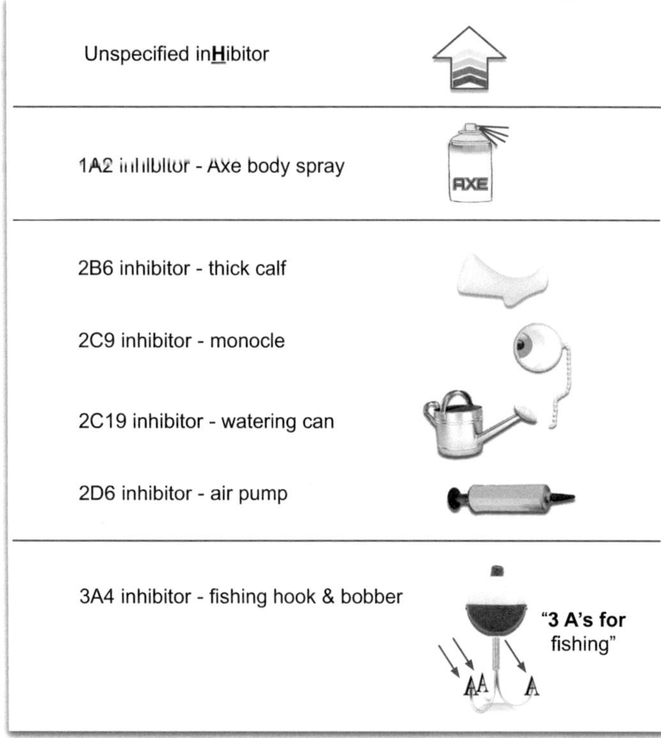

The magnitude to which an in**H**ibitor increases the serum concentration of a specific substrate depends on the number of alternative pathways available to metabolize the substrate. If the drug is a substrate of, e.g., 1A2, 2D6 *and* 3A4, then inhibiting one of the three pathways should be of no consequence. Such substrates may be described as multi-CYP.

For a substrate metabolized by a single pathway, the effect of inhibition (and induction) will be dramatic. An example is lurasidone (Latuda), which is contraindicated with strong 3A4 inhibitors or inducers.

Some inhibitors are stronger than others. In general, expect blood levels of susceptible substrates to increase in the ballpark of:

- mild inhibitor ~ 25% - 50% increase
- moderate inhibitor ~ 50% - 100% increase
- strong inhibitor > 100% increase

Expect these numbers to vary widely between substrates and individuals, often unpredictably.

The "**flu**ffers" – notorious strong in**H**ibitors:

- **fluvoxamine** (Luvox) - SSRI
- **fluoxetine** (Prozac) - SSRI
- **fluconazole** (Diflucan) - antifungal
- **ketoconazole** (Nizoral) - antifungal

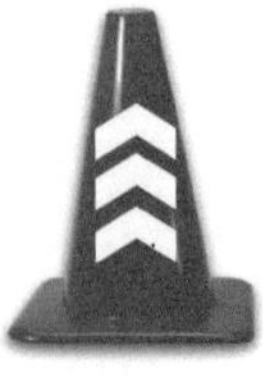

The last two are "cone"-azole antifungals.

ENZYME INDUCTION

The opposite of in**H**ibition is **inDuction**. In**D**uction occurs when an in**D**ucer stimulates the liver to produce extra enzymes, leading to enhanced metabolism and quicker clearance of victim drugs. More often than not, an inducer is itself a substrate of the enzyme.

The **D** is for **D**own, i.e., **D**ecreased serum concentrations of victim substrates. Unlike in**H**ibition (**H** for **H**urried), in**D**uction is **D**elayed, not taking full effect for 2 to 4 weeks while we...
wait for the liver to ramp up enzyme production.

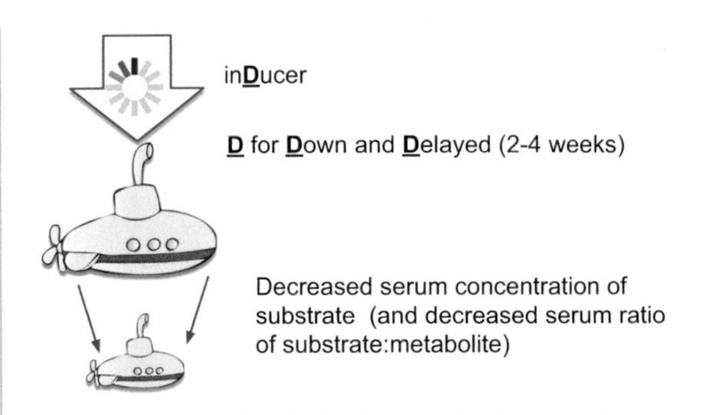

In**D**ucers will be depicted by:

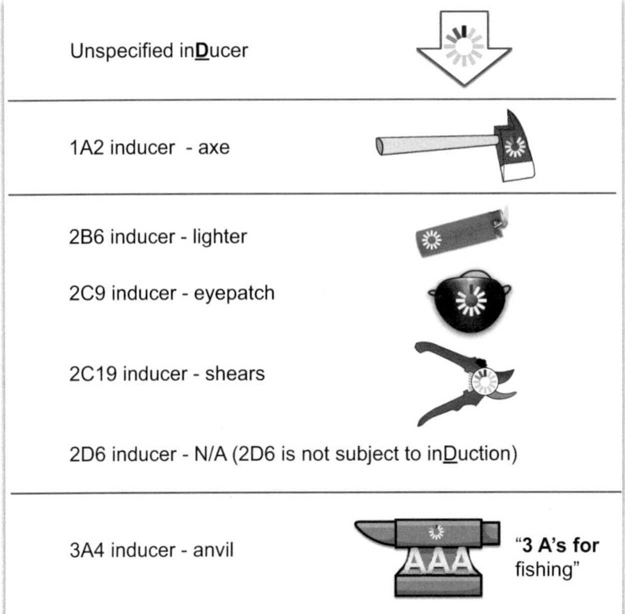

THE SHREDDERS

The **"shredders"** are four **strong inDucers** of several CYPs, which cause countless chemicals to be quickly expelled from the body:

- **carbamazepine** (Tegretol) – antiepileptic
- **phenobarbital** (Luminal) – **barb**iturate
- **phenytoin** (Dilantin) – antiepileptic
- **rifampin** (Rifadin) – antimicrobial

Dr. Jonathan Heldt refers to the shredders as **"Carb & Barb"** in his book *Memorable Psychopharmacology.*

St John's Wort (herbal antidepressant) also in**D**uces several CYPs, but does so with less potency than the four shredders.

Can shredding be problematic even if the patient is not taking a victim medication? Consider this:

Long-term use of a shredder leads to decreased bone mineral density. This is presumably due to in**D**uction of enzymes that inactivate 25(OH) vitamin **D**.

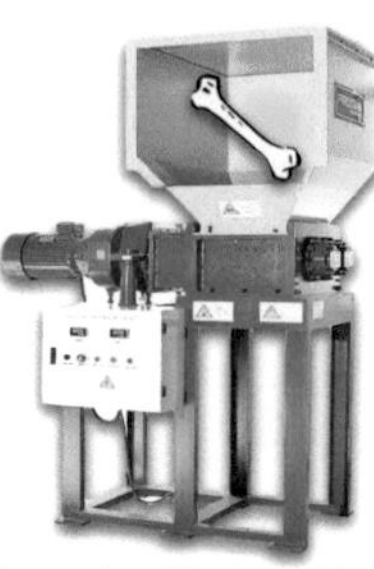
bone shredding machine

REVERSAL OF INHIBITION/ INDUCTION

All things being equal, it is best to avoid prescribing strong inducers or inhibitors. Even if there is no problematic interaction at the time, having a strong inhibitor or inducer on board may complicate future medication management.

Consider an individual on an established medication regimen who stops taking an inducer or inhibitor. The serum concentration of victim substrate(s) will change due to the **reversal** of induction/inhibition.

After an in**D**ucer is withdrawn, the concentration of a victim substrate will increase gradually (**D** for **D**elayed) over a few weeks because the extra CYP enzymes are degraded without being replenished.

When an in**Hi**bitor is stopped, levels of a victim substrate will decrease as soon as the aggressor exits the body. "**H**urriedly" does not mean immediately, because it takes about **five half-lives** for a drug to be completely cleared.

For a patient on several psychotropic medications, reversal of inhibition or induction can really throw things out of whack.

While ePrescribe systems may warn the doctor when starting an interacting medication, there will be **no warning** when stopping a medication will lead to a reversal situation.

An example of **reversal of inDuction** involves tobacco, which is a 1A2 in**D**ucer. A patient taking clozapine (1A2 substrate) stops smoking, reversing in**D**uction and causing clozapine levels to potentially double over the first week (which is faster than occurs with other inducers). The individual may become obtunded, hypotensive, or even have a seizure. To avoid this, the recommendation is to decrease clozapine dose by 10% daily over the first four days upon smoking cessation, and to check clozapine blood levels before and after the dose adjustment. Note that nicotine products (gum, patches, e-cigs) do not induce 1A2.

Consider a patient taking alprazolam (Xanax, 3A4 substrate) who suddenly stops **flu**voxamine (Luvox, 3A4 in**H**ibitor). In absence of the inhibitor, alprazolam levels drop (from double) to normal. Since fluvoxamine has a short elimination half-life of 15 hours, it should be out of the body at 75 hours (15 hr x 5). So, you would expect the patient on Xanax to become more anxious 3 days after stopping Luvox. It may be difficult to discern whether the patient's emerging distress is due to serotonin withdrawal or decreased alprazolam levels.

Although reversal of in**H**ibition is typically faster than reversal of induction, this does not apply to inhibitors with extremely long half-lives. For instance, **flu**oxetine (Prozac) has a long elimination half-life of about 7 days, keeping itself around for about 35 days (7 days x 5). Consider a patient with schizophrenia on aripiprazole (Abilify, 2D6 substrate) who stops Prozac (2D6 in**H**ibitor). The patient is doing well at one month, but becomes paranoid two months out. Unless the prescriber anticipated this possibility, no one will realize what happened.

PRODRUGS

Phase I metabolism typically involves biotransformation of an active drug to an inactive (or less active) chemical.

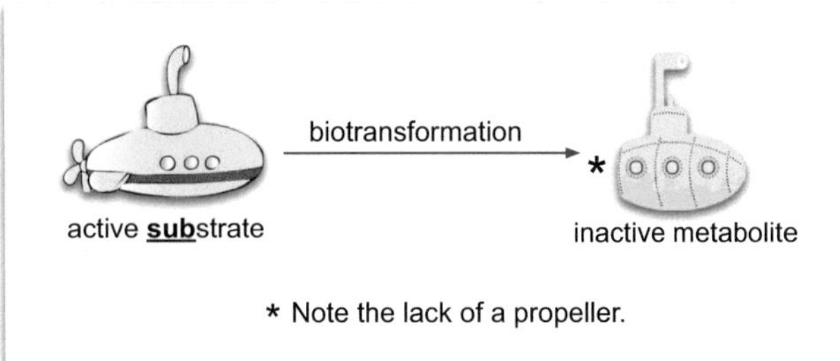

For a few medications, the parent drug has low therapeutic activity until it is biotransformed by a CYP enzyme. In such cases, the substrate is called a **prodrug**, and the biotransformation process can be referred to as **bioactivation**.

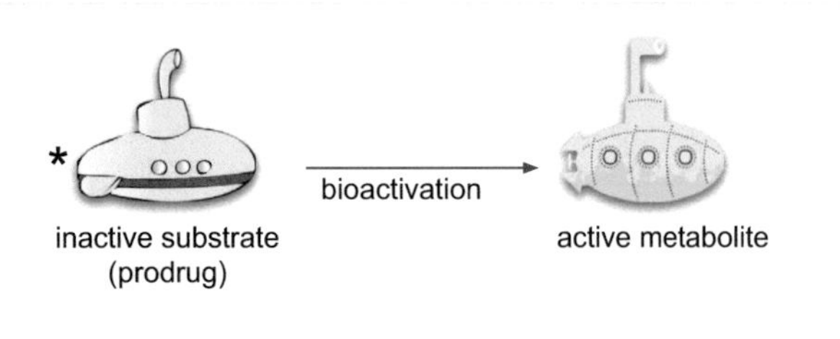

For most medications (active parent drug to inactive metabolite) in**D**uction decreases (**D** for **D**own) effect of the drug and in**H**ibition (**H** for **H**igh) amplifies the therapeutic effect and/or side effects.

With prodrugs, the opposite effect is observed clinically. Induction increases and inhibition decreases the medication's effect(s).

Don't let prodrugs confuse you. In**H**ibitors increase and In**D**ucers decrease the levels of substrate regardless of whether the parent drug is pharmacologically active.

The following are **prodrugs** activated by 2D6:

- **Codeine** – metabolized to morphine
- **Tramadol** (Ultram) – weak opioid
- **Tamoxifen** – anti-estrogen for breast cancer

The bowling ball is explained on page 15.

PHASE II METABOLISM

Phase II metabolism occurs in the liver and is subject to kinetic interactions. CYP enzymes are not involved.

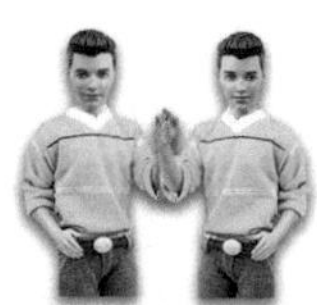

Two Kens without a bottle to "CYP" (sip)

Phase II reactions typically involve **conjugation** of a substrate with **glucuronic acid**. This makes it water soluble and prepped for renal excretion.

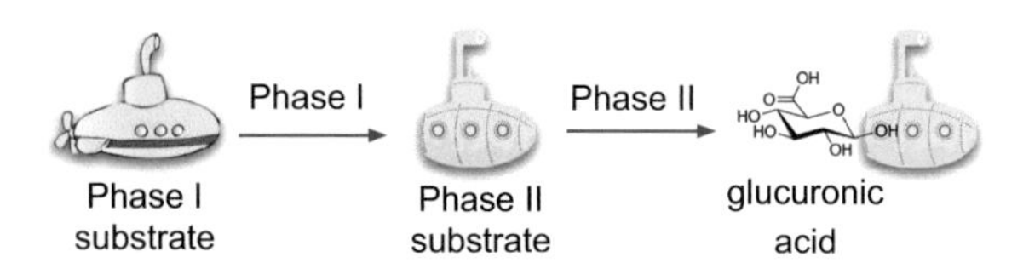

The responsible enzyme is UDP-glucuronosyltransferase, abbreviated **UGT**, as in "U Got Tagged" with glucuronic acid.

Medications metabolized primarily by Phase II are relatively immune to drug interactions. Examples of clinically relevant Phase II interactions are those involving lamotrigine (Lamictal) as a substrate, as featured on page 17.

RENAL CLEARANCE

A few medications are excreted in urine without being metabolised. Such drugs are not subject to Phase I or II interactions, but may be victims of kinetic interactions. Renal "aggressors" act by slowing or hastening the rate of excretion of the victim drug in urine.

Interactions affecting renal clearance of victim drugs are also considered (pharmaco)"Ken"etic.

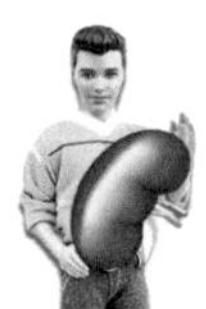

The aggressor in a renal interaction is not referred to as an inducer or inhibitor, because no enzyme is involved. Nor is the victim called a substrate, because it is not being biotransformed.

Lithium, excreted unchanged in urine, is subject to victimization as illustrated on page 26.

CYP GENETIC PROFILES

Genetic polymorphisms can influence an individual's medication kinetics, which is most relevant for 2D6 and 2C19. Let's talk about 2D6, arguably the most consequential example.

Most individuals are genetically equipped with 2D6 genes that produce normal 2D6 enzymes that metabolize 2D6 substrates at the usual rate. These normal individuals are said to have a 2D6 **extensive metabolizer** (EM) genotype, resulting in a 2D6 EM phenotype.

Here is a cute representation of how a normal individual, i.e., 2D6 **extensive metabolizer** (EM), processes 2D6 substrates. The air inside the beach ball represents the substrate, which is being expelled from the ball as metabolite at the usual rate. 2D6 substrates will have typical elimination half-lives.

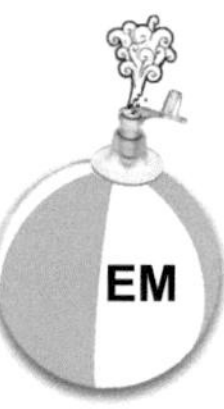

About 5% of the population have extra copies of 2D6 genes, resulting in an **ultrarapid metabolizer** (UM) phenotype. These individuals clear 2D6 substrates quickly.

For 2D6 **ultrarapid metabolizers** (UM), the air (2D6 substrate) flows out of the ball quickly as metabolite. 2D6 substrates could be ineffective for these individuals (with the exception of 2D6 prodrugs, which could be be too strong).

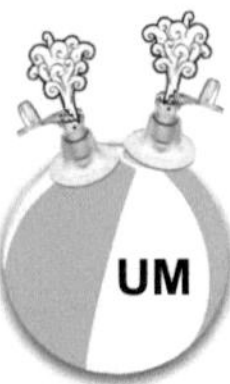

About 10% of individuals have defective 2D6 enzymes resulting in a 2D6 **poor metabolizer** (PM) phenotype. This condition may be found on a diagnosis list as "Cytochrome P450 2D6 enzyme deficiency".

For 2D6 "**POOR ME**"tabolizers (PM), air accumulates, resulting in unexpectedly long half-lives for 2D6 substrates. These individuals are more likely to report side effects.

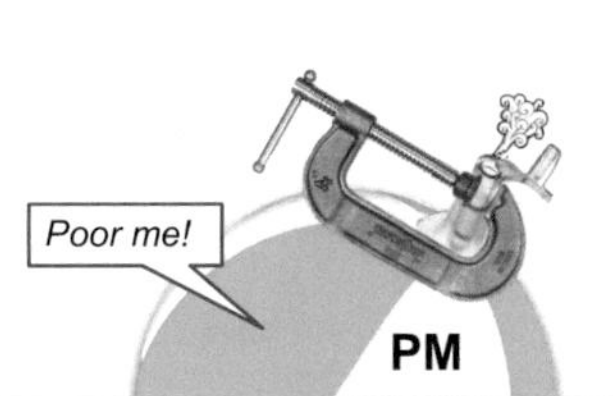

An individual taking a strong 2D6 in**H**ibitor (pump as illustrated on page 15) will metabolize 2D6 substrates **as if** the individual had a 2D6 PM genotype.

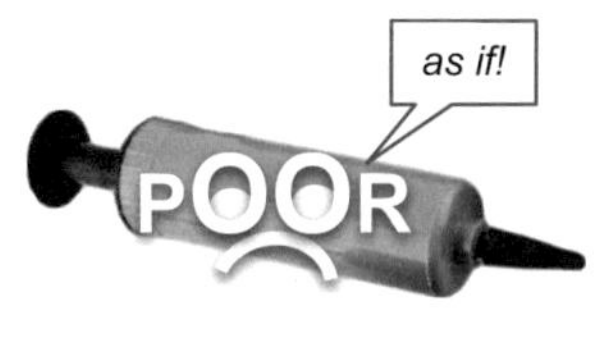

In summary, genetic testing of CYP polymorphisms will interpret the metabolizer profile for a given enzyme as either:

- Extensive metabolizer (EM) – normal
- Ultrarapid metabolizer (UM) – fast clearance of substrates
- Poor metabolizer (PM) – slow clearance of substrates

A genetic test result of **intermediate metabolizer** (IM) means that enzyme activity is likely to be a bit lower than that of an EM, i.e., an intermediate between EM and PM. Generally, IM individuals can be clinically managed normally, like an EM individual.

Standalone 2D6 genotyping costs at least $200. GeneSight or Genecept panels cost about $4,000 and report the six relevant CYPs and two UGT enzymes (UGT1A4 and UGT2B15). 23andMe ($199) reports 1A2, 2C9, and 2C19, among 100s of other genes. 23andMe does not report the most relevant CYP genotype, 2D6, because the genetics of 2D6 metabolism is more complicated.

Genotyping may be useful when choosing which medication to prescribe an individual patient. With GeneSight, about 1 in 5 patients have a genetic variation relevant to their treatment. For an individual already established on a medication, serum drug levels may be more useful than genotyping. There are situations when knowing the actual blood levels of clozapine, risperidone, olanzapine, aripiprazole, haloperidol, lamotrigine, etc. are clinically relevant. Unfortunately, these tests usually must be sent to an outside lab, and it may take a week to see the results. Levels of lithium, carbamazepine, and valproic acid are usually reported the same day.

P-GLYCOPROTEIN

P-glycoprotein (P-gp) is a gatekeeper at the gut lumen and the blood-brain barrier. P-gp pumps P-gp substrates out of the brain—"Pumpers gonna pump".

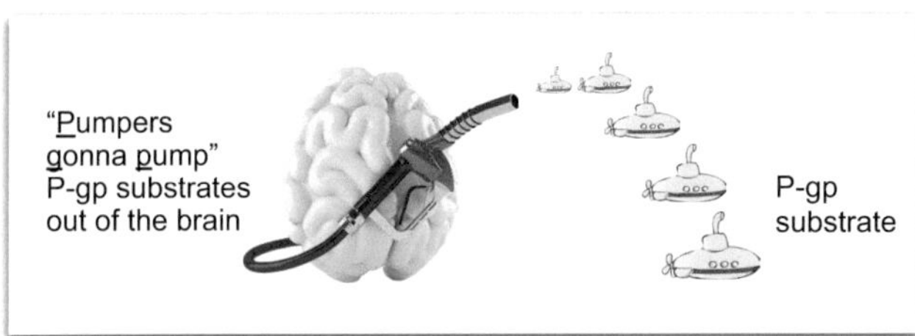

An example of a relevant P-gp interaction involves the OTC opioid antidiarrheal loperamide (Imodium). Loperamide does not cause central opioid effects under normal circumstances. If the individual takes a potent P-gp inhibitor, megadose loperamide can stay in the brain long enough to cause euphoria. The P-gp inhibitor typically used the achieve this recreational effect is omeprazole (Prilosec).

THE NATURE OF THIS INFORMATION

The information presented in the remainder of this chapter is a synthesis of numerous sources including Lexicomp, Flockhart Table, ePocrates, Carlat Medication Fact Book, Stahl's Essential Psychopharmacology, The Medical Letter, Current Psychiatry, GeneSight, Genecept, various research papers and FDA prescribing information for the individual drugs.

Reputable sources are often at odds with each other regarding the strength of specific inducers/inhibitors, the vulnerability of specific substrates to induction/inhibition, or even which CYPs are relevant to a specific medication. CYP interactions are continuously being discovered and clarified. Even with the freshest information and full knowledge of a patient's genotype, the magnitude of a specific CYP interaction is difficult to predict.

HOW TO APPLY THIS INFORMATION

Refer to the tables on pages 20 and 21. Highlight the medications that you prescribe. First acquaint yourself with the in**D**ucers because the list is short. Memorize the bolded inducers (shredders) and those that you highlighted. After you know the inducers, move to the in**H**ibitor column. Memorize the bolded inhibitors (fluffers) and your highlighted medications. Mood stabilizers, antiepileptics, barbiturates and benzodiazepines are already highlighted for you in this edition of *Cafer's Psychopharmacology*.

When it comes to substrates, memorization is less important. Substrates are only relevant when an inducer or inhibitor is on board, or if the patient has a special metabolizer genotype. Of the medications you prescribe, be aware of the more susceptible substrates.

Consider running an interaction check whenever a patient is taking a shredder, fluffer, systemic antifungal, HIV medication, or cancer medication. ePocrates.com and the ePocrates app are adequate, and free.

Keep things simple. When choosing new medications, avoid major inducers and inhibitors if suitable alternatives are available. For the complicated psychiatric patient on several medications, try to avoid carbamazepine (shredder inducer) and the **flu**ffer SSRIs (**flu**oxetine and **flu**voxamine). Among SSRIs, escitalopram (Lexapro) and sertraline (Zoloft) are good choices - they are 2C19 substrates but do not induce or inhibit.

Also think about choosing less vulnerable substrates. Each drug on pages 18 and 19 is depicted in box/bubble because it is generally not involved in clinically significant kinetic interactions (although dynamic interactions almost always apply). You don't have to worry much about benzodiazepine interactions if you stick to the "LOT" benzos—lorazepam, oxazepam and temazepam. Most antipsychotics are susceptible substrates, but not so much for ziprasidone, loxapine and paliperidone.

This book uses picture association as a memorization technique. Pages 10 through 17 establish a visual mnemonic framework for various kinetic interactions that will be reinforced by a "mascot" for each drug. The mascots serve a double purpose of helping you remember trade name / generic name pairings.

Since you probably won't be mentioning CYP nomenclature in casual conversation, you might want to bypass the technical naming system altogether. Instead of keeping a list of "3A4 substrates" in your memory bank, you could just learn the school of "fish".

I hope this book empowers you to understand and memorize topics that are otherwise daunting, so you can to use your knowledge to improve patient care. Without further ado, let's start our journey to becoming a superhero of psychotropic medication management.

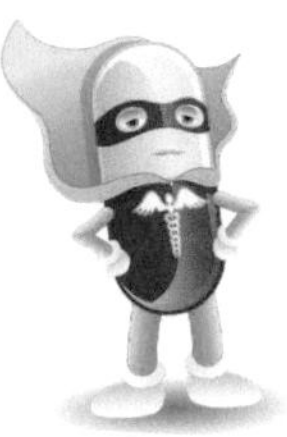

1A2 accounts for 10 - 15% of CYP activity in the liver

Cytochrome P450 1A2 (CYP1A2)

"One Axe to Grind; One Axe to Grow"

52% of individuals are 1A2 ultrarapid metabolizers; < 1% are poor metabolizers

"**1** **A**xe to **2** Grind"

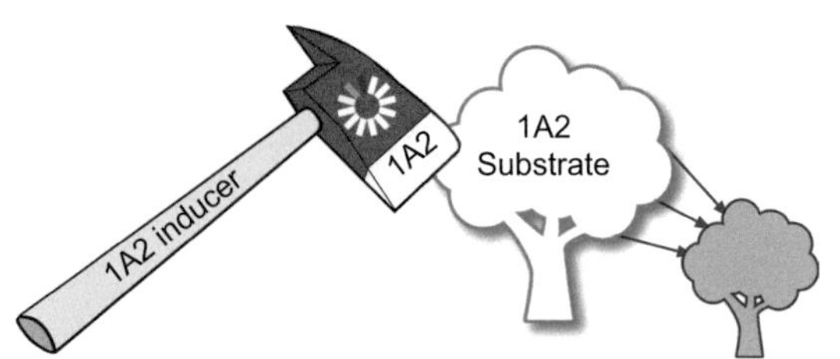

in**D**ucer = **D**own

Decreased substrate levels

induction onsets and reverses slowly = **D**elayed *

Hydrocarbons from smoked herbs such as tobacco and cannabis are moderate potency 1A2 inducers. All other 1A2 inducers are weak.

"**1** **A**xe **2** Grow"

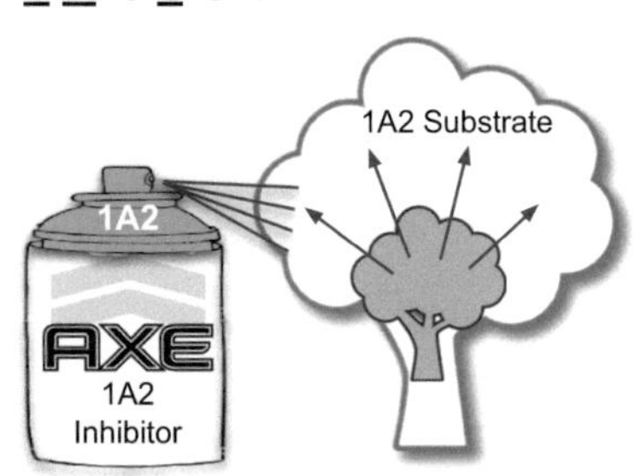

in**H**ibitor = **H**igh

Increased substrate levels

in**H**ibition happens within **H**ours = **H**urried and reverses as soon as the inhibitor is cleared from the body (five half-lives of the inhibitor)

Fluvoxamine (Luvox) is the only strong 1A2 inhibitor.

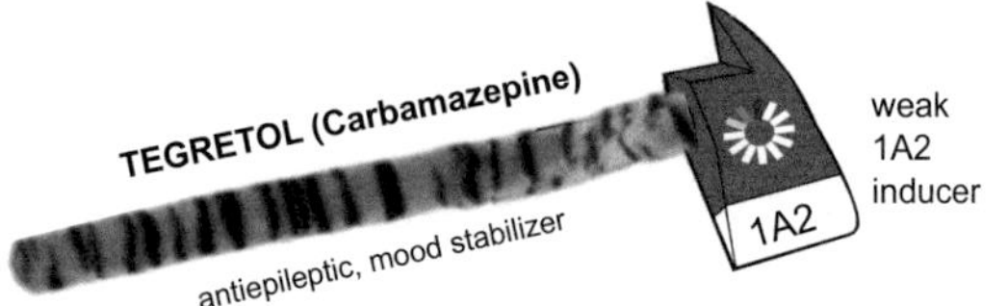

weak 1A2 inducer

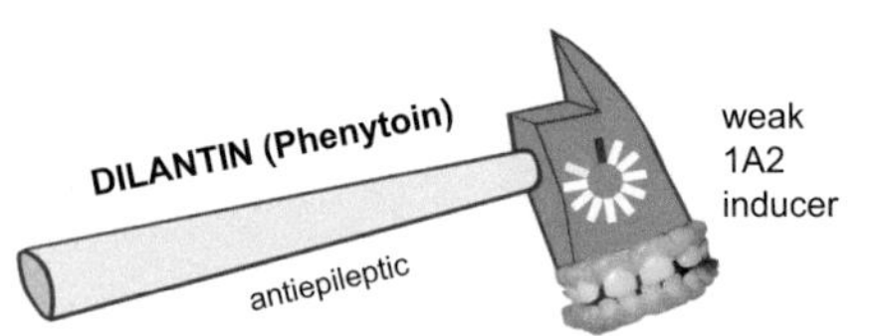

weak 1A2 inducer

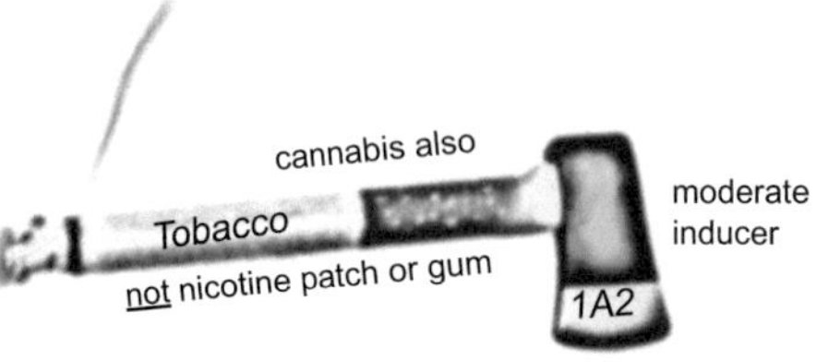

moderate inducer

* Induction by smoking takes about 3 days to start—notice the ax has no spinning wheel like the other axes. Upon cessation of smoking, induction reverses over the first week. This is much faster than with other inducers. 10 cigarettes daily is sufficient for maximum induction effect.

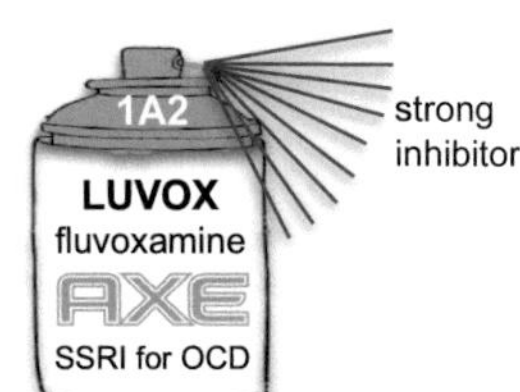

strong inhibitor

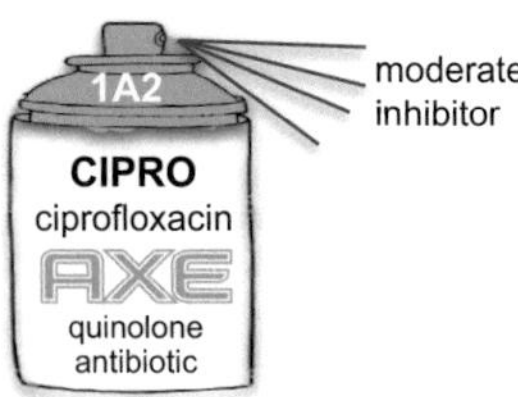

moderate inhibitor

1st Generation Antipsychotics | 2nd Gen Antipsychotics "-pine" trees | Antidepressant

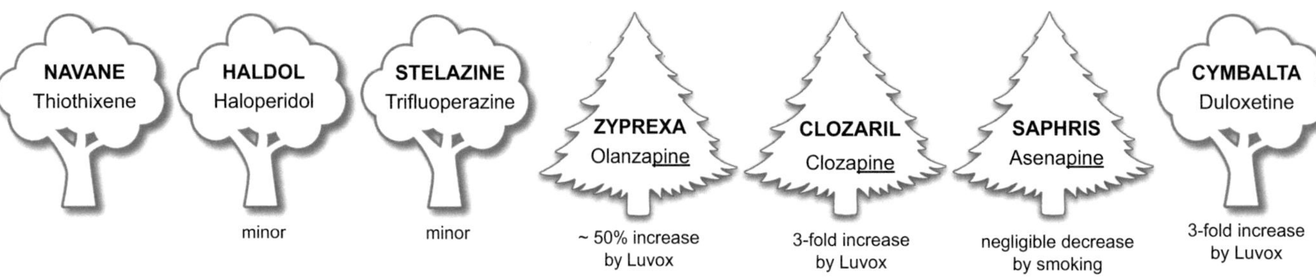

Melatonin agonists

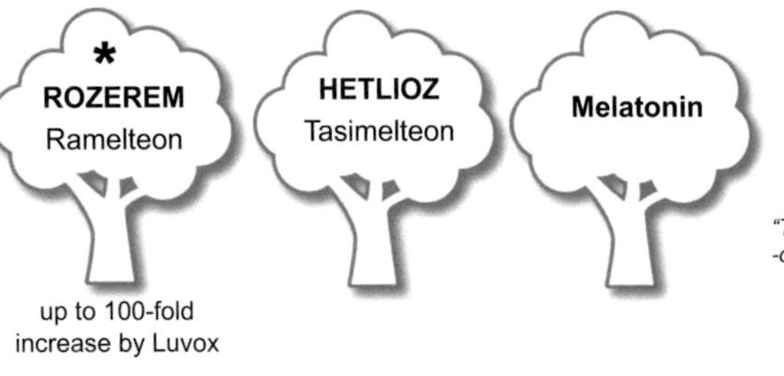

Methylxanthines

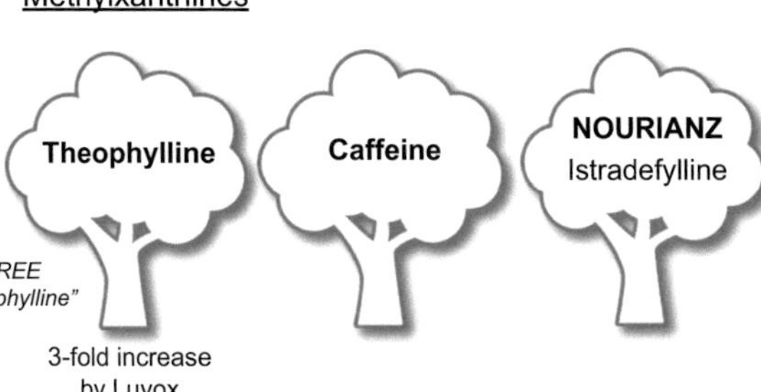

Spasmolytic

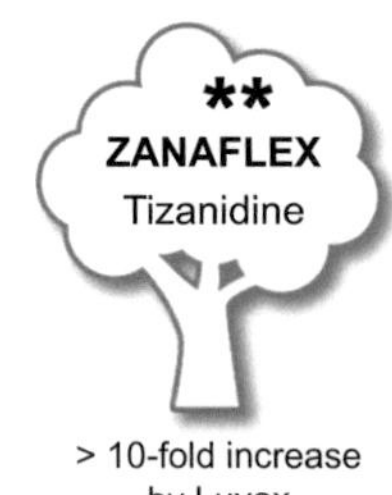

* Contraindicated with Luvox

** Contraindicated with Luvox or Cipro

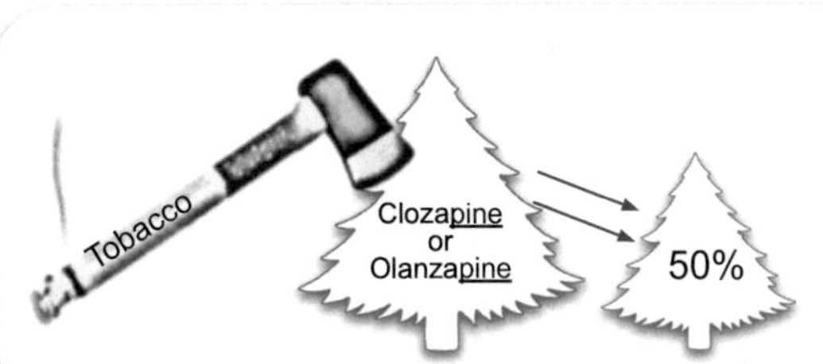

Tobacco **decreases** blood levels of these two "pine trees" by about 50%.

Conclusion: Keep in mind that 52% of individuals have a 1A2 ultrarapid metabolizer genotype, and everyone who smokes has a rapid metabolizer phenotype. The effect of smoking on olanzapine and clozapine is worthy of memorization. Memorization of other 1A2 substrates is of lower priority, as long as you remember to refer to this list whenever Luvox is in the mix. Run an interaction check on any medication regimen that includes Luvox. Try to keep Luvox out of the mix entirely—it is nonessential for treatment of OCD because other SSRIs are equally effective at high doses.

Ciprofloxacin, a moderate 1A2 in**H**ibitor, increases clozapine levels about 2-fold.

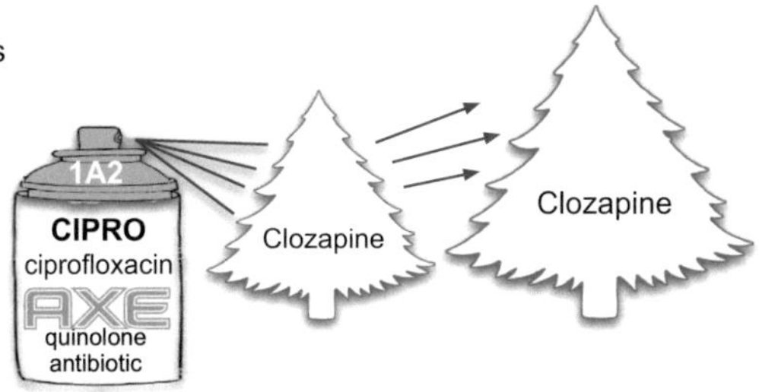

Fluvoxamine, a strong 1A2 in**H**ibitor, increases clozapine levels 3-fold on average, but up to 10-fold in some cases.

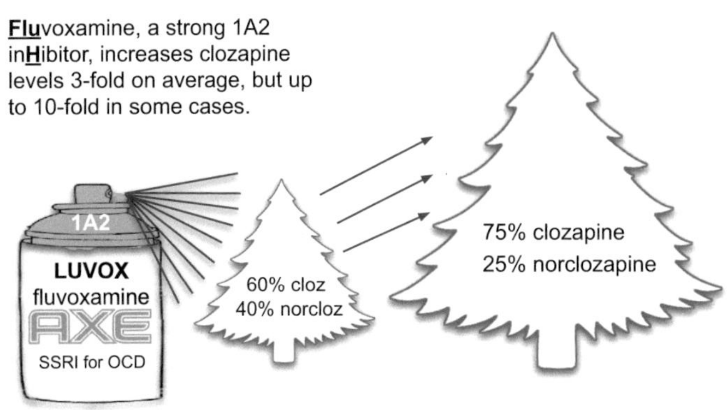

Kinetic interactions can be more complicated than simply increasing/decreasing concentrations of victim substrates.

Combining clozapine and fluvoxamine is hazardous, but can potentially be used for therapeutic advantage. Close monitoring of serum **clozapine levels** would be required.

Norclozapine is the main metabolite of clozapine, formed by 1A2. When clozapine blood levels are reported, clozapine and metabolite (norclozapine) levels are provided separately. Through 1A2 in**H**ibition, Luvox increases the **clozapine:norclozapine ratio**. A **H**igher serum clozapine:norclozapine ratio is generally considered desirable*. Norclozapine provides little antipsychotic benefit and causes weight gain, diabetes, seizures, and neutropenia.

Patients given clozapine 100 mg + Luvox 50 mg daily (compared to clozapine 300 mg monotherapy) demonstrated more improvement with less weight gain. Clozapine levels were similar for both groups with, as expected, lower norclozapine levels for those taking Luvox.
(Lu ML et al, 2018; randomized controlled trial, N=85).

*The negative aspect of a **H**igher clozapine:norclozapine is greater anticholinergic burden (pages 161-162). Clozapine is anticholinergic, whereas norclozapine is cholinergic. Consequently, clozapine causes constipation, while norclozapine does not. The anticholinergic properties of clozapine may impair cognition, whereas norclozapine provides cognitive benefits such as enhanced working memory.

Certain physiologic states may increase levels of olanzapine and clozapine up to 2-fold.

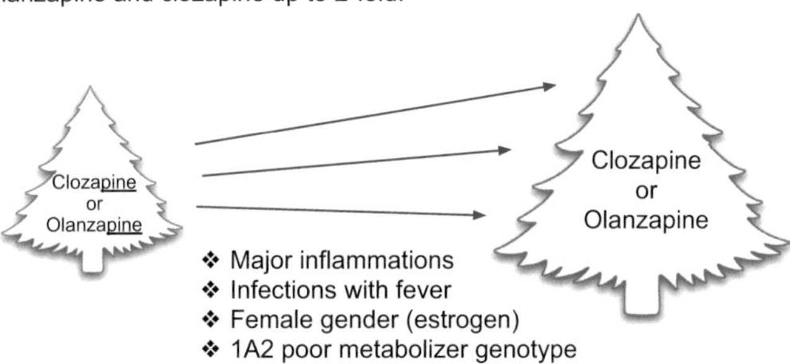

- Major inflammations
- Infections with fever
- Female gender (estrogen)
- 1A2 poor metabolizer genotype

For a patient with efficacy or tolerability issues, consider monitoring serum levels of the antipsychotic. The author checks clozapine levels routinely, and olanzapine levels in some cases.

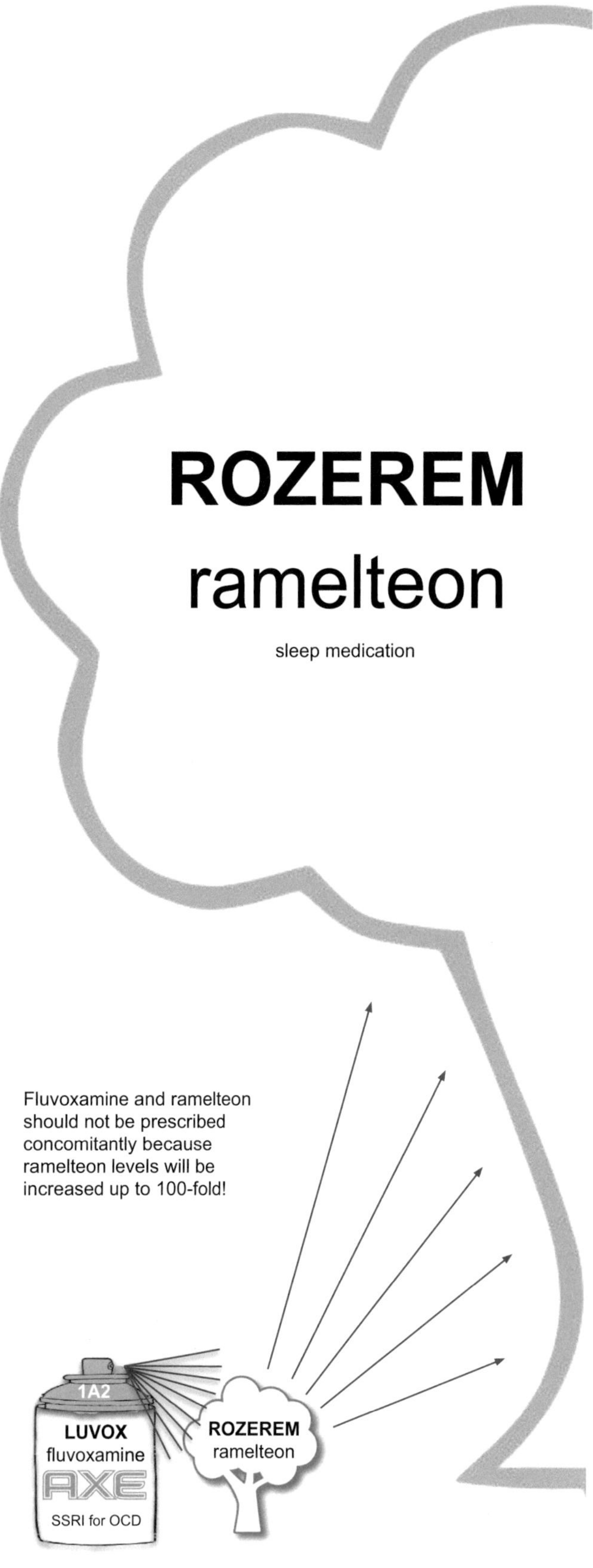

Fluvoxamine and ramelteon should not be prescribed concomitantly because ramelteon levels will be increased up to 100-fold!

Cytochrome P450 2B6 (CYP2B6)

"Tube Socks"

3% of individuals are 2B6 ultrarapid metabolizers; 7% are poor metabolizers

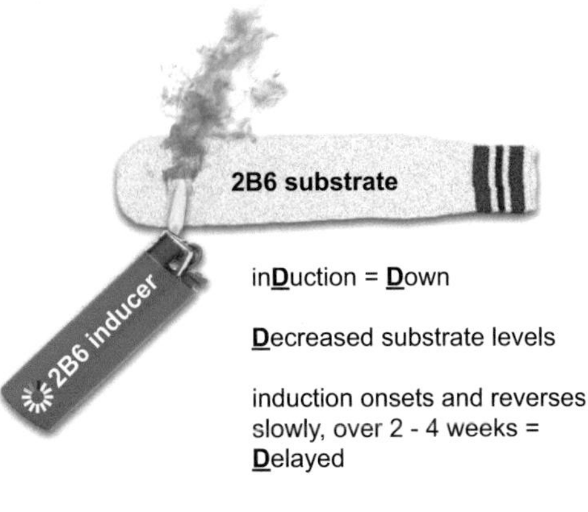

inDuction = Down

Decreased substrate levels

induction onsets and reverses slowly, over 2 - 4 weeks = Delayed

There are no strong 2B6 inducers.

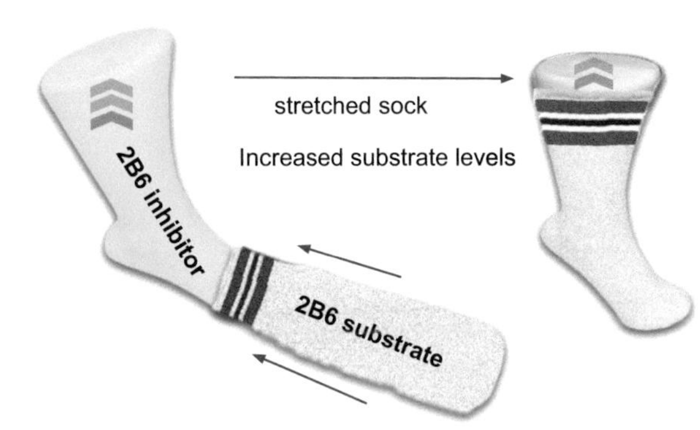

inHibition = High

inHibition happens within Hours = Hurried and reverses as soon as the inhibitor is cleared from the body (five half-lives of the inhibitor)

There are no strong 2B6 inhibitors.

Carbamazepine
TEGRETOL

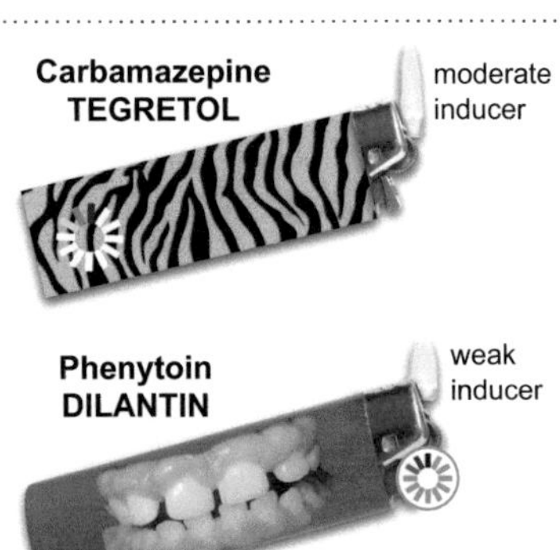

moderate inducer

Phenytoin
DILANTIN

weak inducer

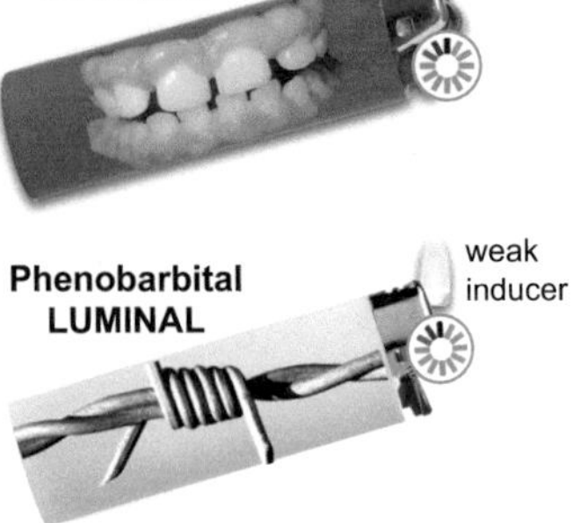

Phenobarbital
LUMINAL

weak inducer

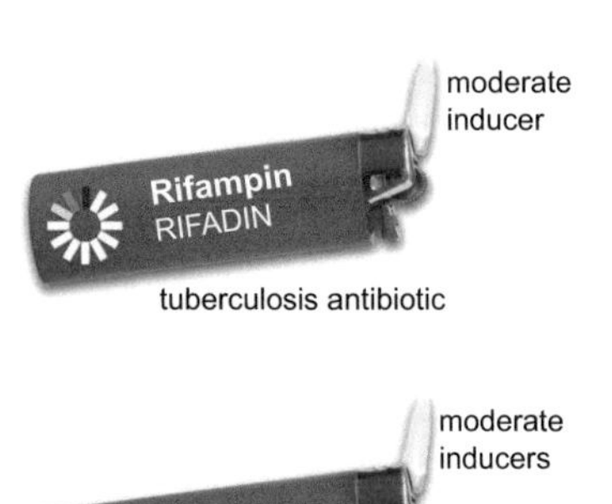

moderate inducer

tuberculosis antibiotic

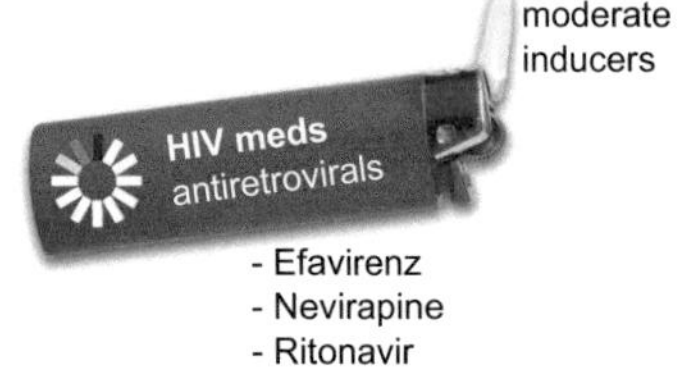

moderate inducers

- Efavirenz
- Nevirapine
- Ritonavir

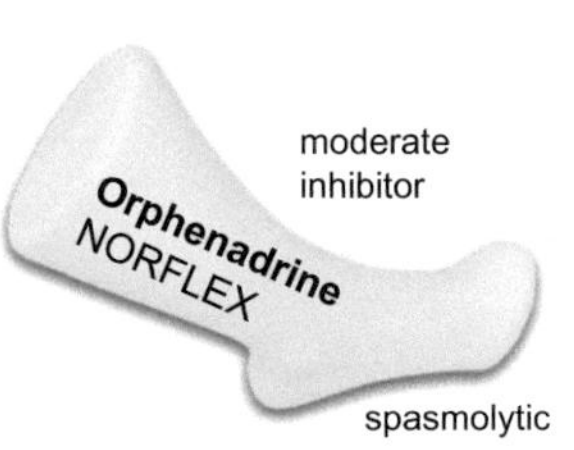

moderate inhibitor

spasmolytic

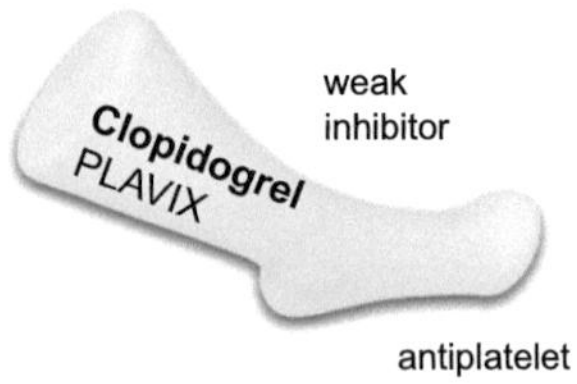

weak inhibitor

antiplatelet

Antidepressants

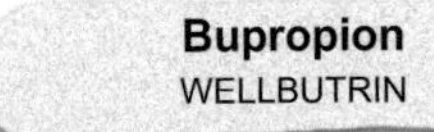

also 2D6 for -OH metabolite

NDRI

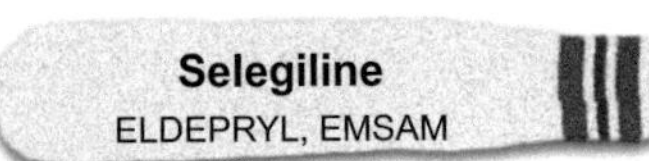

MAOI

Alkylating Drugs for Cancer

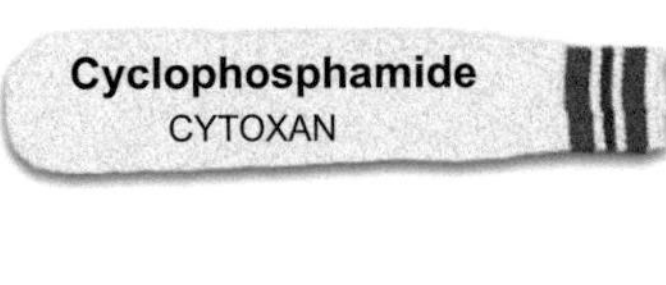

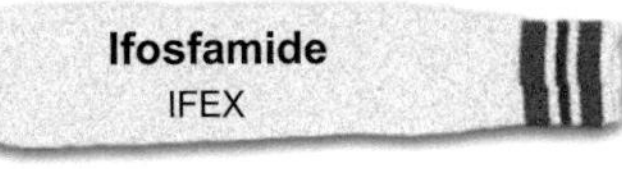

Opioid

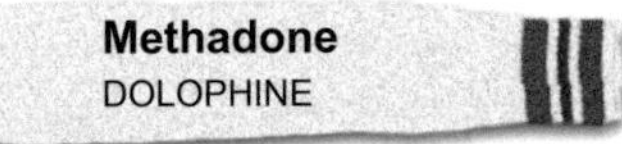

3% of the population are 2B6 ultrarapid metabolizers (UMs). Methadone efficacy for these individuals will be poor, and their methadone drug screen may be negative.

Anaesthetics

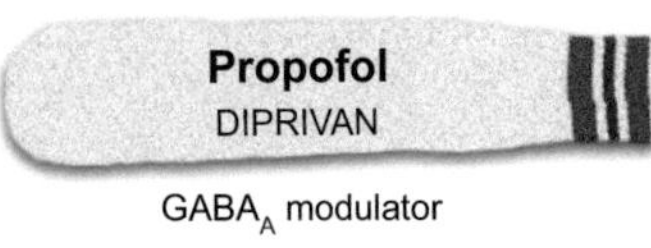

$GABA_A$ modulator

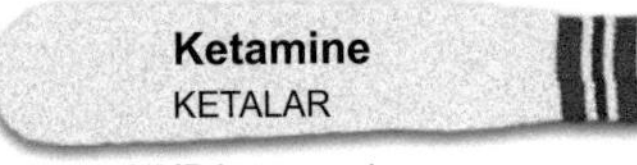

NMDA antagonist

Esketamine
SPRAVATO

NMDA antagonist

NNRTIs for HIV

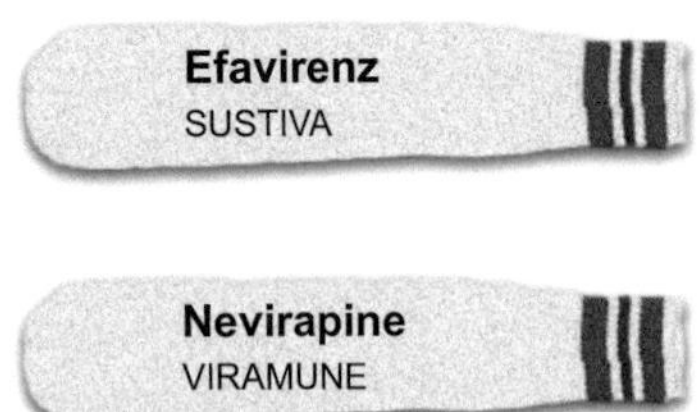

Conclusion: Fortunately, there are no strong inhibitors or inducers of 2B6. For psychiatrists, 2B6 is of minimal significance, unless methadone is being prescribed (see above). You will want to run an interaction check (e.g., ePocrates or Lexicomp) whenever a medication regimen includes a shredder, cancer medication, HIV medication, or systemic antifungal.

For psychiatry, 2C9 interactions are of little clinical significance.

Cytochrome P450 2C9 (CYP2C9)

"To See Nice(ly)"

0% of individuals are 2C9 ultrarapid metabolizers; 5% are poor metabolizers

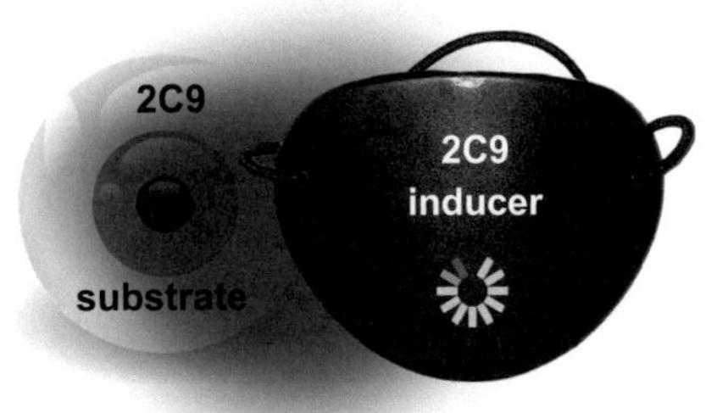

inDuction = Down

Decreased substrate levels

induction onsets and reverses slowly, over 2 - 4 weeks = Delayed

There are no strong 2C9 inducers.

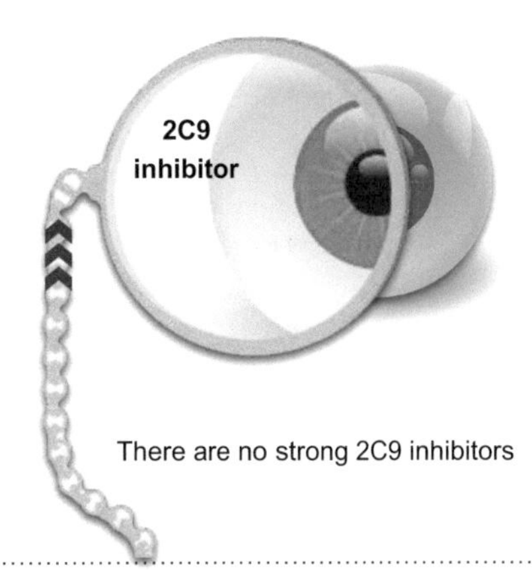

inHibition = High

Increased substrate leve

inHibition happens within Hours = Hurried

Inhibition reverses as soon as the inhibitor is cleared from the body (five half-lives of the inhibitor)

There are no strong 2C9 inhibitors

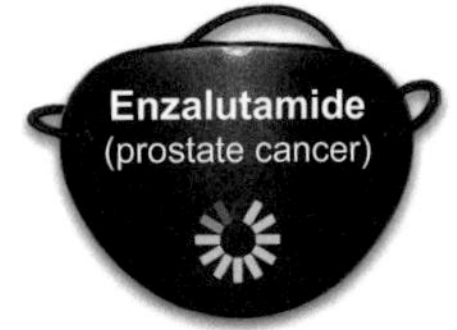

moderate inducer

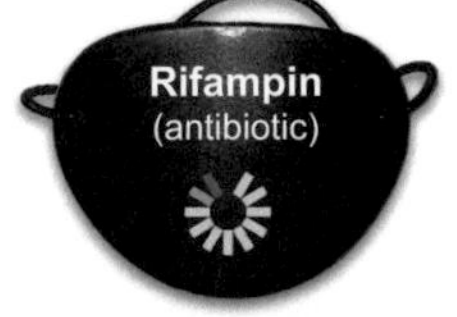

moderate inducer

LUMINAL
Phenobarbital

weak inducer

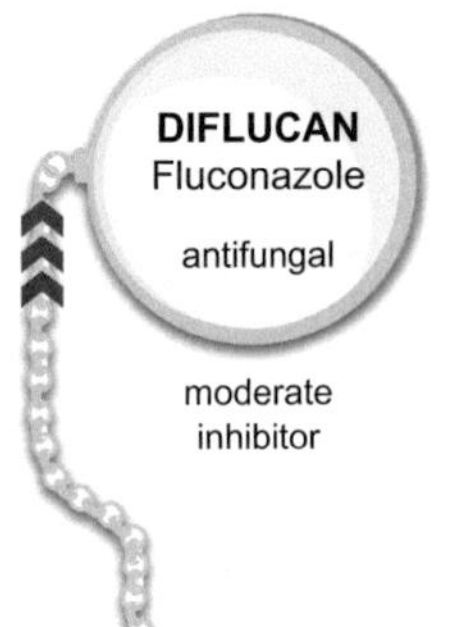

moderate inhibitor

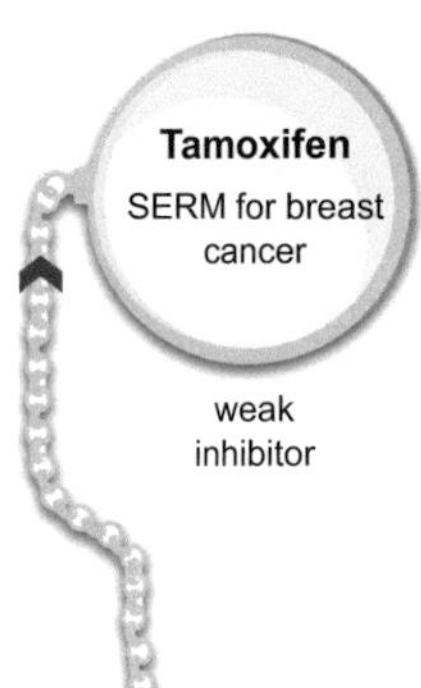

weak inhibitor

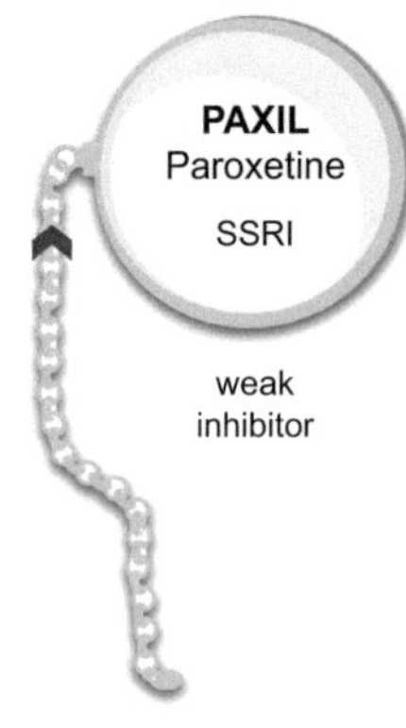

weak inhibitor

Antiepileptics

DILANTIN

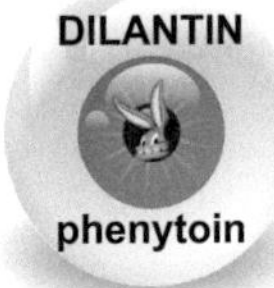

phenytoin

"d-EYE-lantin; phen-EYE-toin"

Also 2C19

DEPAKOTE

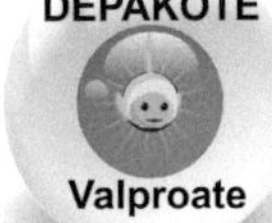

Valproate

"Dep-EYE-kote"

2C9 contributes only 25% to the metabolism of VPA

Anticoagulant

COUMADIN

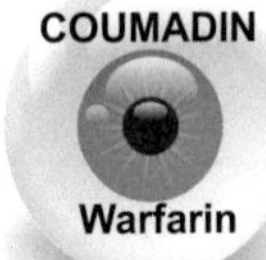

Warfarin

"coum-EYE-din"

Also 2C19

Sulfonylureas for DM

MICRONASE

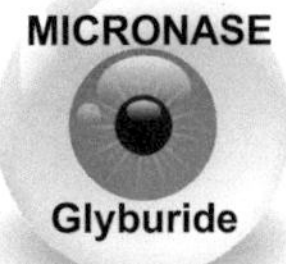

Glyburide

"glybur-EYED"

AMARYL

Glimepiride

"glimepir-EYED"

GLUCOTROL

Glipizide

"Glipiz-EYED"

ORINASE

Tolbutamide

"tolbutam-EYED"

ARB for HTN

COZAAR

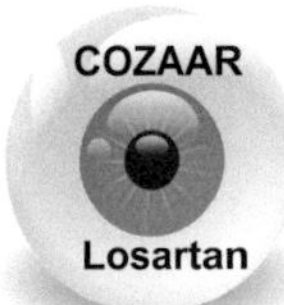

Losartan

"Coz-EYEr"

Also 3A4

Lipid lowering

LESCOL

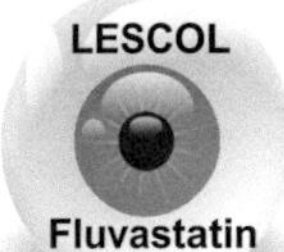

Fluvastatin

"fluv-EYE-statin"

Libido enhancer

ADDYI

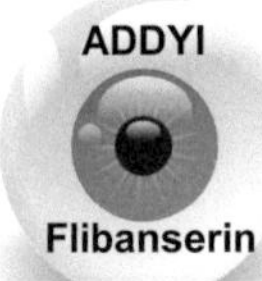

Flibanserin

NSAID

FELDENE

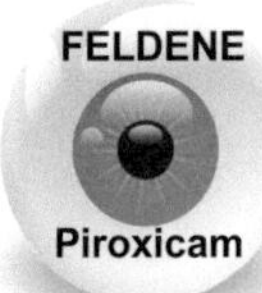

Piroxicam

"p-EYE-roxicam"

COX-2 inhibitor

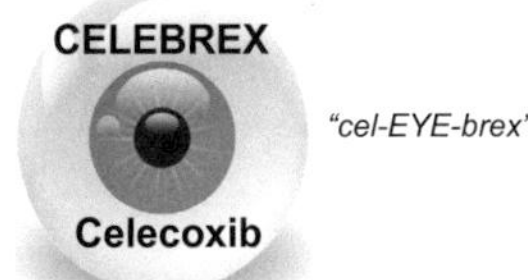

Conclusion: Valproic acid (VPA) is the only psychotropic medication involved in 2C9 interactions. Check VPA levels more often if the patient is taking enzalutamide, rifampin or diflucan; but don't expect much variance from baseline.

Cytochrome P450 2C19 (CYP2C19)

"To See Nice Things (grow)"

10% of individuals are 2C19 ultrarapid metabolizers; 5% are poor metabolizers

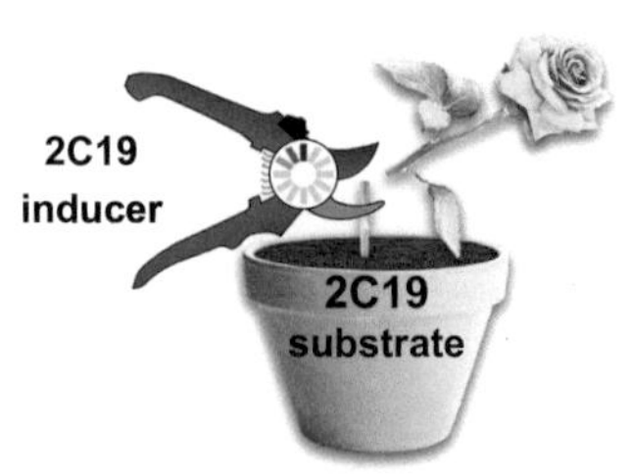

in**D**uction = **D**own

Decreased substrate levels

induction onsets and reverses slowly, over 2 - 4 weeks = **D**elayed

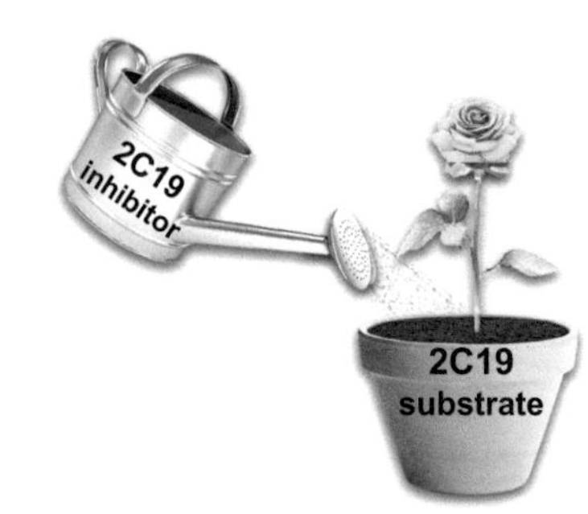

in**H**ibition = **H**igh

Increased substrate levels

in**H**ibition happens within **H**ours = **H**urried

Inhibition reverses as soon as the inhibitor is cleared from the body (five half-lives of the inhibitor)

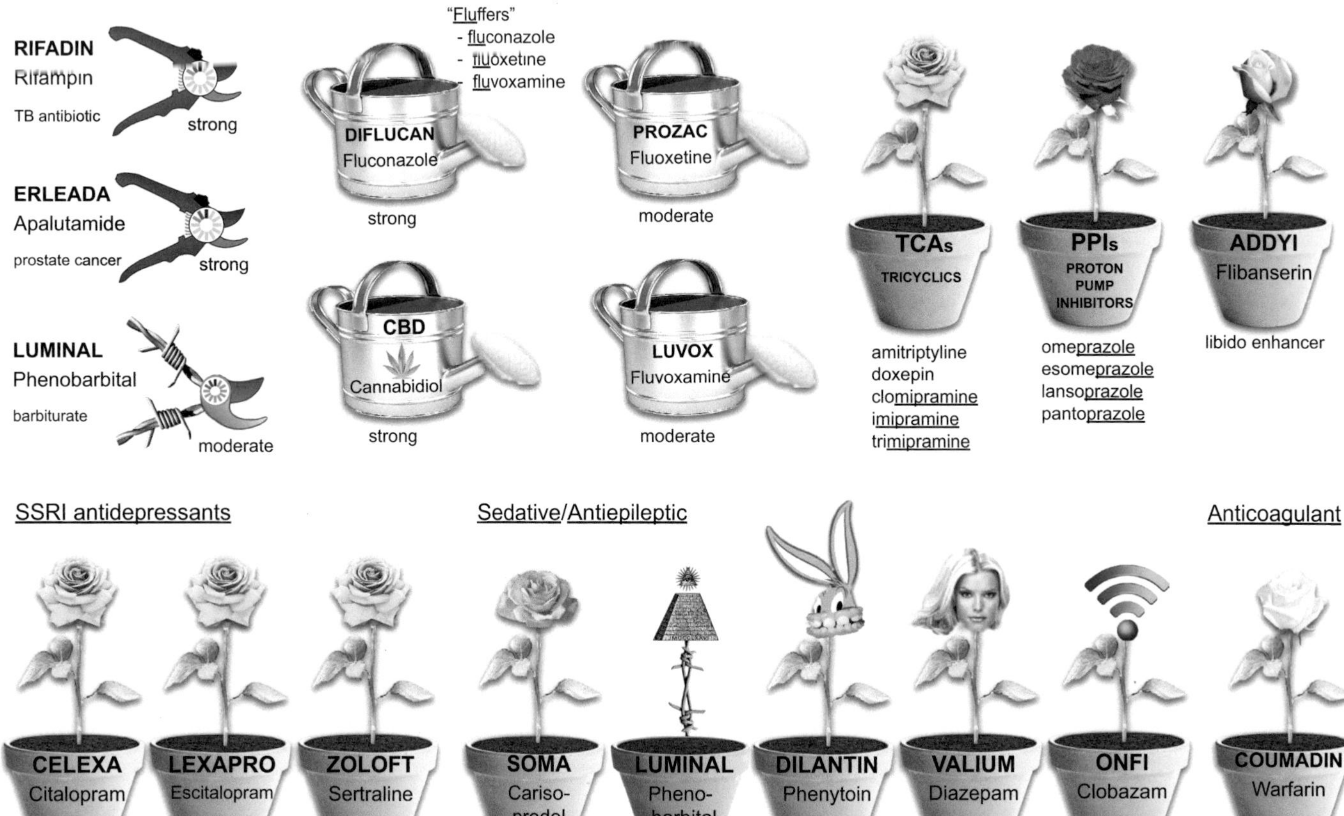

2C19 poor metabolizers (PM)

Individuals with a 2C19 PM genotype clear 2C19 substrates slowly, leading to **H**igher blood levels (as if they were taking a 2C19 in**H**ibitor). Standard doses of 2C19 substrates may be too strong.

* 2C19 poor metabolizers should not exceed 20 mg of citalopram (QT prolongation).

5% of population (20% of Asians)

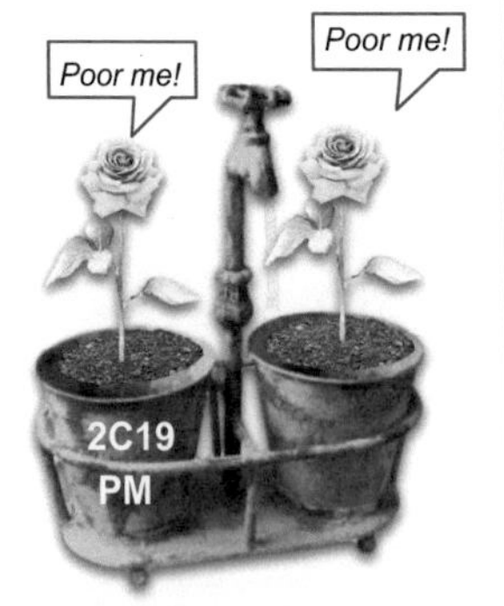

2C19 ultrarapid metabolizers (UM)

2C19 UM individuals clear 2C19 substrates quickly, leading to low blood levels. These individuals are more likely to be non-responders to 2C19 substrates.

10% of population

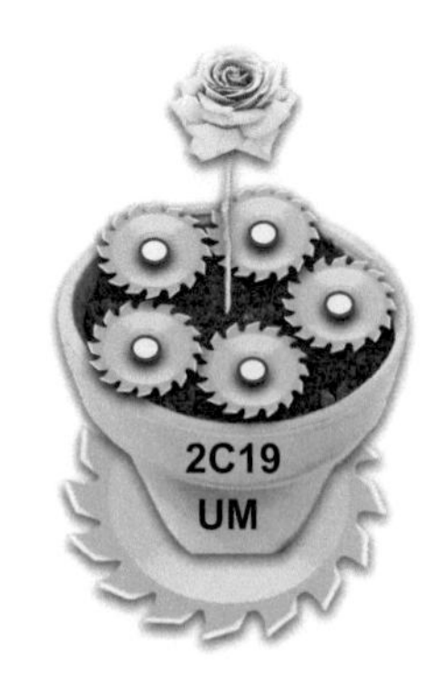

Conclusion: 2C19 genotyping is not typically ordered as a standalone test, but if 2C19 metabolizer genotype is known (e.g., from GeneSight or Genecept), the information can be put to good use when dosing (es)citalopram and sertraline. Knowledge of metabolizer status is not essential because these SSRIs can be titrated the old-fashioned way, according to response and side effects. In any event, avoid prescribing Soma, Valium, or phenobarbital for anxiety due to their particularly high risk of abuse and dependence. Avoid St. John's Wort due to interactions, and because it only works for mild depression.

2D6 metabolizes ~ 12% of prescription drugs. Notice how all of the -oxetine's are 2D6 inhibitors and/or substrates.

Cytochrome P450 2D6 (CYP2D6)

"Too Darn Sexy"

5% of individuals are 2D6 ultrarapid metabolizers (UM).
10% are poor metabolizers (PM).

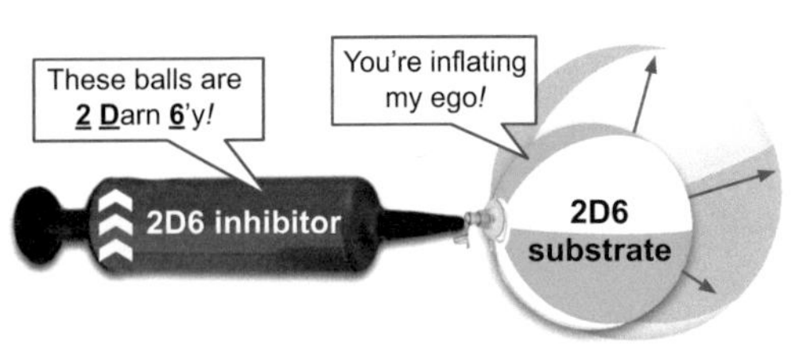

2D6 enzymes cannot be induced.

in**H**ibition = **H**igh

Increased substrate levels

in**H**ibition happens within **H**ours = **H**urried

Inhibition reverses as soon as the inhibitor is cleared from the body (five half-lives of the inhibitor)

Prodrugs are substrates that are less potent than their metabolites. Ordinary substrates (beach balls) are deactivated by 2D6. Prodrugs (bowling balls) are *activated* by 2D6. In the presence of an inhibitor prodrugs are less effective.

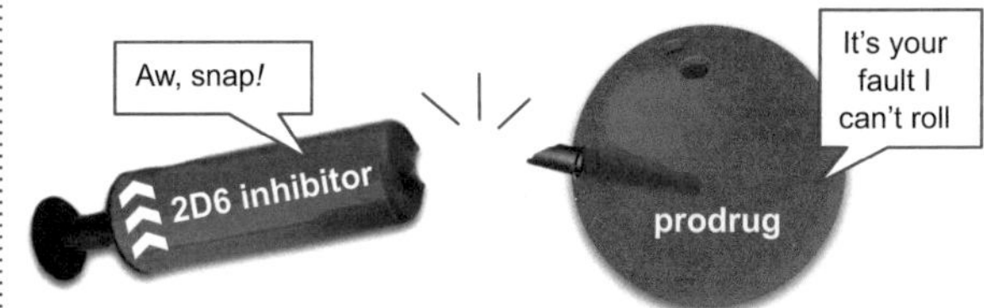

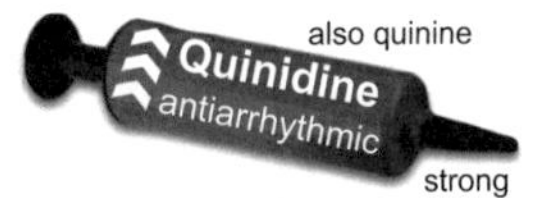

also quinine

strong

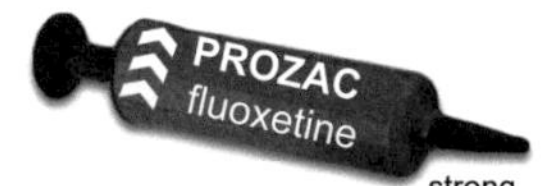

strong

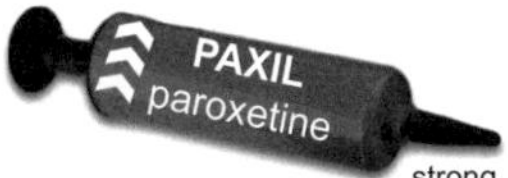

strong

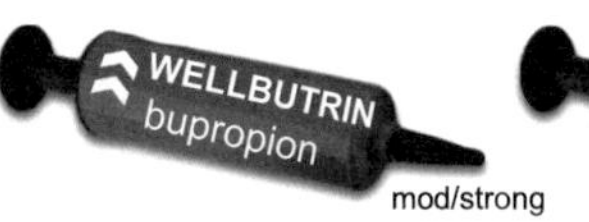

mod/strong

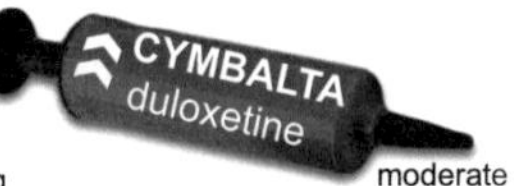

moderate

Antidepressants

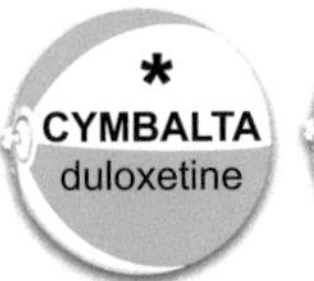

SNRI

* STRATTERA atomoxetine

SNRI for ADHD

* TRINTELLIX vortioxetine

SPARI

OH-bupropion

active metabolite of bupropion (Wellbutrin)

* Tricyclics TCAs

especially:
amoxapine
protriptyline
(nortriptyline)
(desipramine)

VMAT inhibitors

AUSTEDO Deutetrabenazine

also tetrabenazine

Antitussive

DXM dextromethorphan

Anti-HTN

LOPRESSOR metoprolol

beta blocker

1st Gen Antipsychotics (FGA)

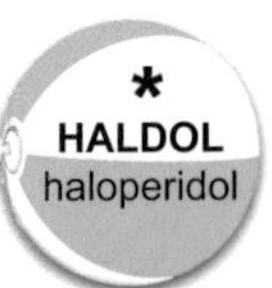

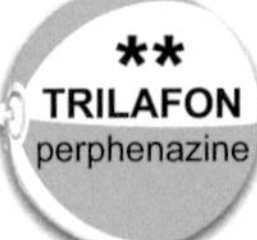

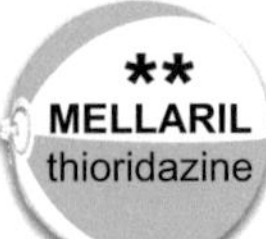

** ORAP pimozide

2D6 genotyping required

2nd Gen Antipsychotics (SGA)

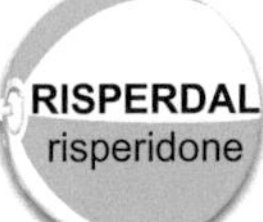

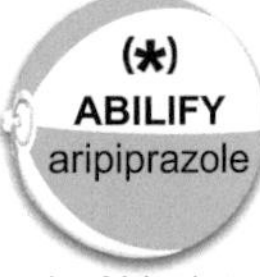

also 3A4 substrate

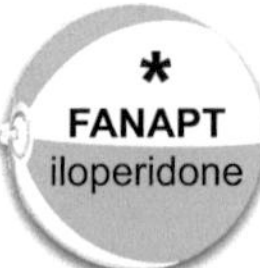

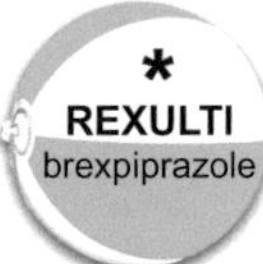

Pro-drugs

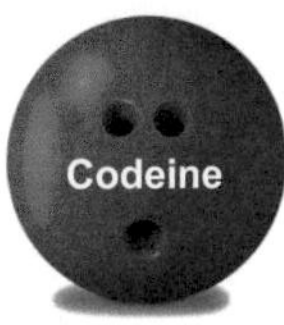

metabolized to morphine

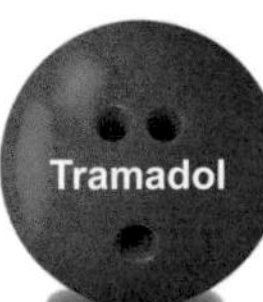

weak opioid and SNRI

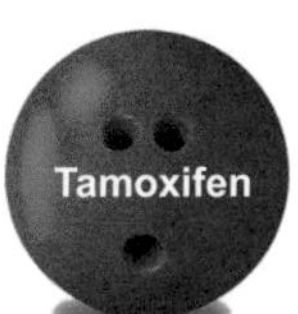

breast cancer

2D6 poor metabolizers have defective 2D6 enzymes. Substrates are cleared slowly (by other pathways) or are unmetabolized leading to **H**igher blood levels, **as if** the patient were taking an in**H**ibitor.

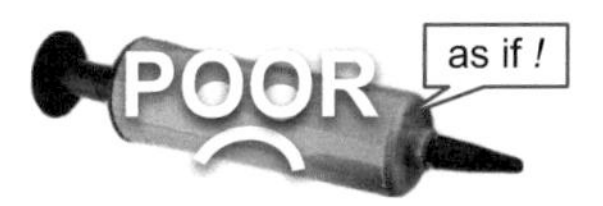

** 2D6 genotyping is recommended prior to starting these medications, which are increased 3- to 4-fold with 2D6 PMs. Mellaril is contraindicated for 2D6 PMs.

* 50% dose reduction is recommended for 2D6 poor metabolizers

(*) According to the label, use 75% of Abilify dose if 2D6 PM. Use 50% Abilify dose if 2D6 PM and taking a 3A4 inhibitor.

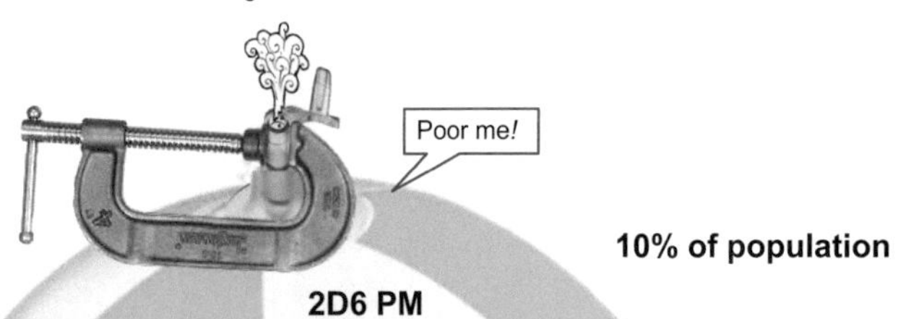

10% of population

2D6 extensive metabolizers have the typical genotype and process 2D6 substrates as expected

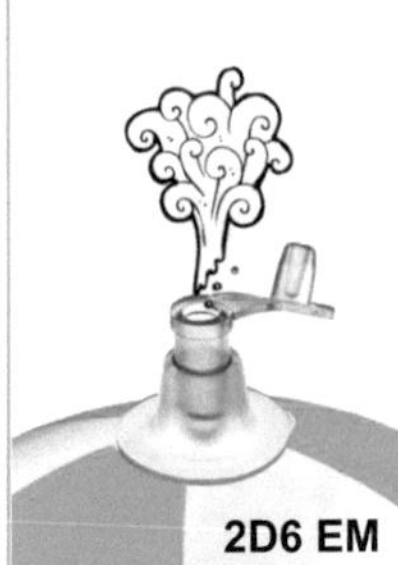

2D6 **ultrarapid metabolizers** clear 2D6 substrates quickly. These individuals are more likely to be non-responders to 2D6 substrates (excluding 2D6 prodrugs, which may be too strong). Relatively common among those with Middle Eastern or North African heritage.

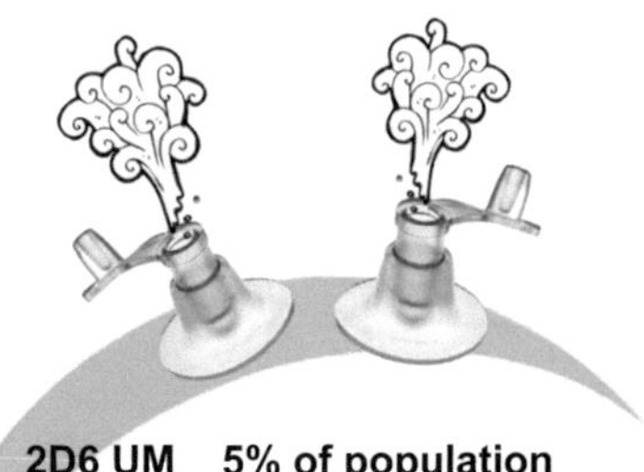

5% of population

Conclusion: 2D6 interactions need to be understood by prescribers of antidepressants and antipsychotics. To avoid 2D6 interactions, use Lexapro or Zoloft instead of Prozac/Paxil. Consider Invega ($330) instead of Risperdal ($12), although cost is an issue. No anticonvulsants, mood stabilizers or benzodiazepines are involved in 2D6 metabolism.

Among the CYP genetic assays, 2D6 is the most useful. The test is about $200 as a standalone, and is recommended prior to starting Trilafon, Mellaril, or Orap—three antipsychotics that psychiatrists rarely prescribe. For the other 2D6 substrates, serum drug levels may be more useful than genotyping. The author commonly checks blood levels of haloperidol, risperidone and aripiprazole if there are issues with efficacy or tolerability.

> 50% of prescription drugs are 3A4 substrates – plenty of fish!

Cytochrome P450 3A4 (CYP3A4)

"3 A's For (fishing)"

0% of individuals are 3A4 ultrarapid metabolizers; <1% are poor metabolizers

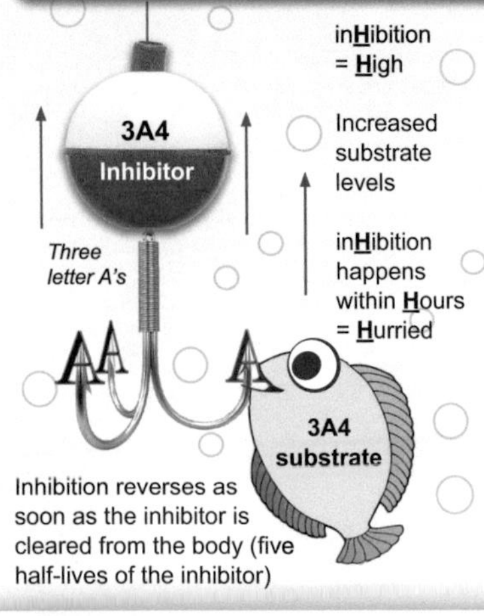

in**H**ibition = **H**igh

Increased substrate levels

in**H**ibition happens within **H**ours = **H**urried

Inhibition reverses as soon as the inhibitor is cleared from the body (five half-lives of the inhibitor)

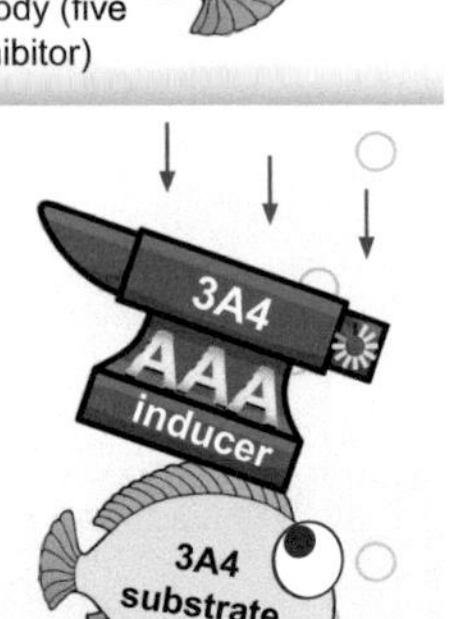

in**D**uction = **D**own

Decreased substrate levels

induction onsets and reverses slowly, over 2- 4 weeks = **D**elayed

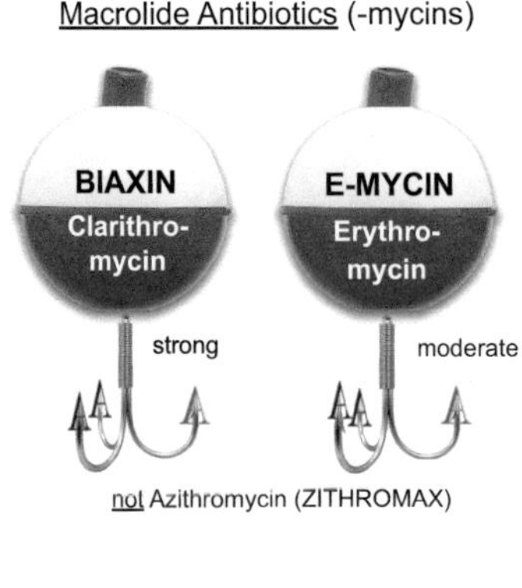
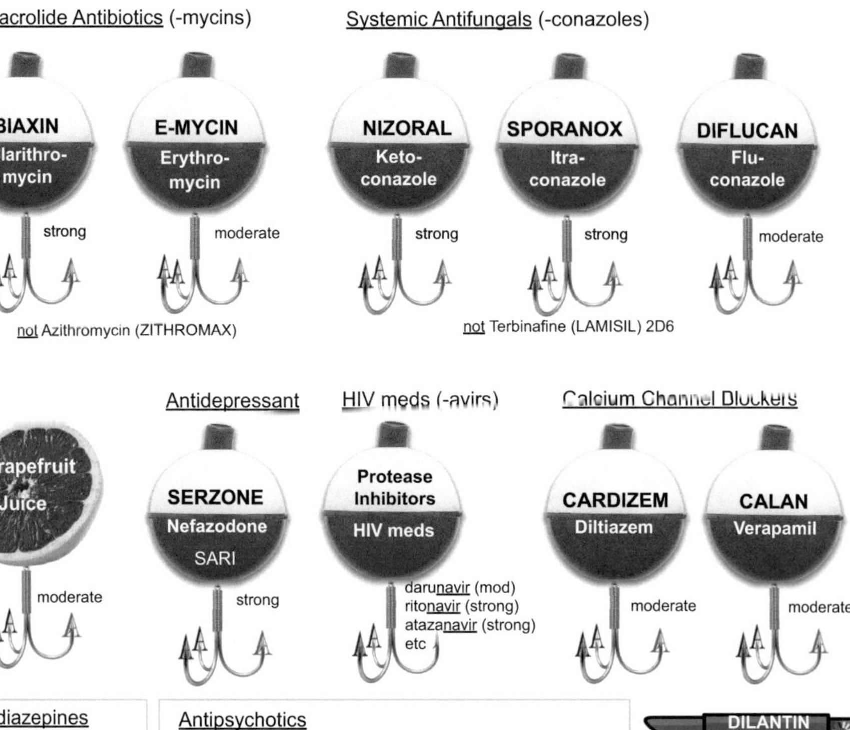

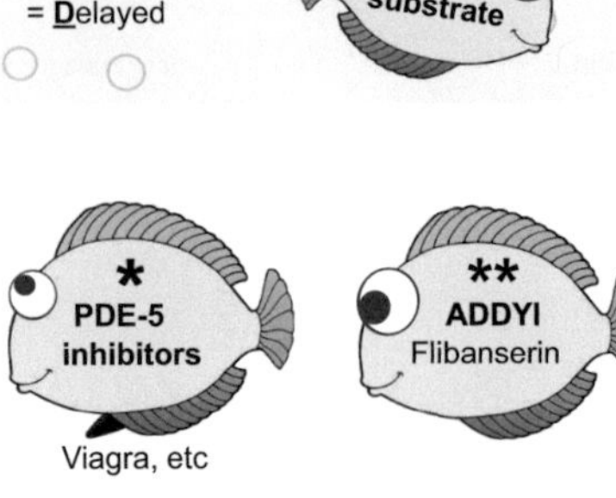

Viagra, etc

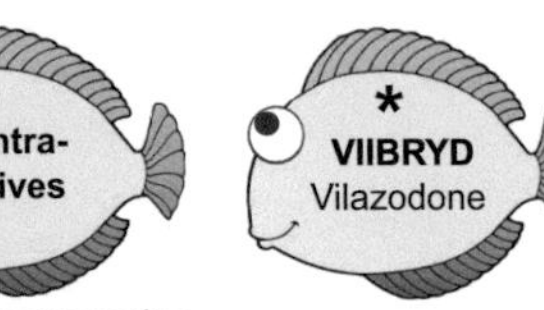

estrogens,progestins

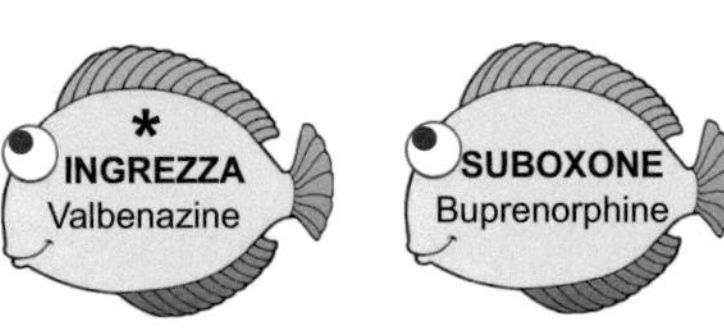

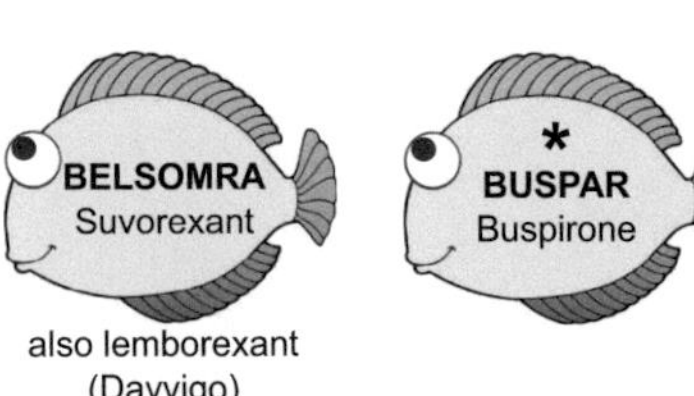

also lemborexant (Dayvigo)

Risk of rhabdomyolysis in combination with 3A4 in**H**ibitors

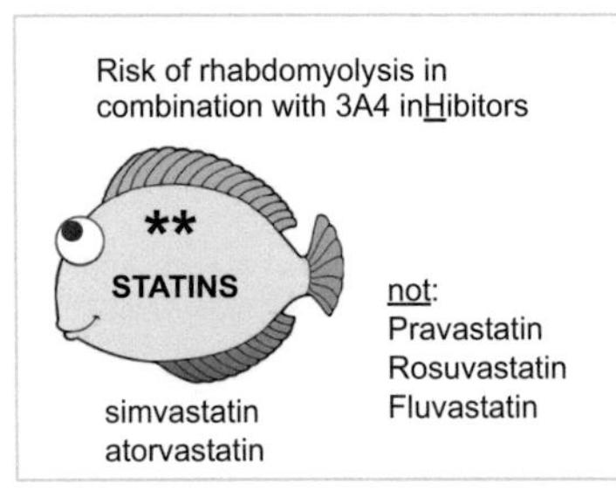

simvastatin
atorvastatin

not:
Pravastatin
Rosuvastatin
Fluvastatin

Benzodiazepines

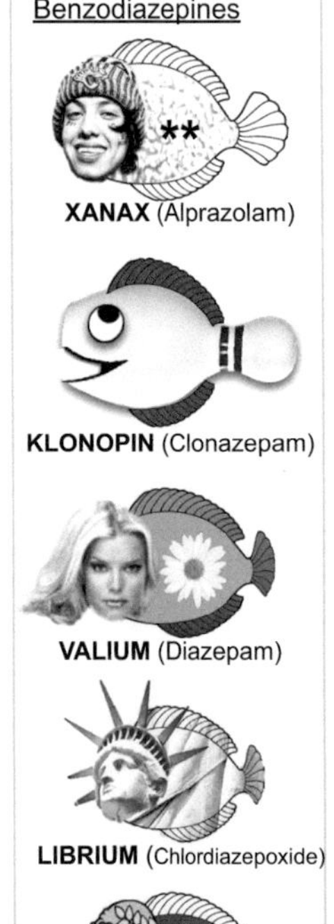
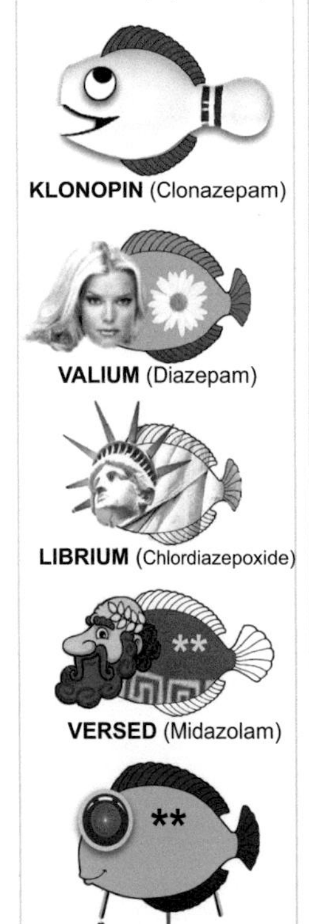
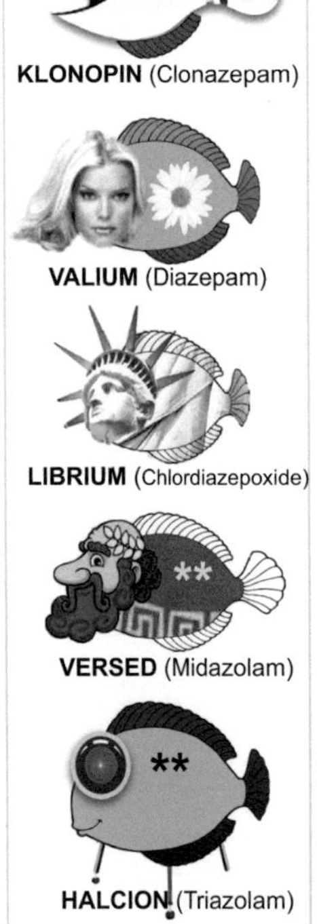

XANAX (Alprazolam) **

KLONOPIN (Clonazepam)

VALIUM (Diazepam)

LIBRIUM (Chlordiazepoxide)

VERSED (Midazolam) **

HALCION (Triazolam) **

also:
Estazolam (Prosom) **
Clorazepate (Tranxene)

not:
Lorazepam (Ativan)
Oxazepam (Serax))
Temazepam (Restoril)
Clobazam (Onfi) 2C19

Antipsychotics

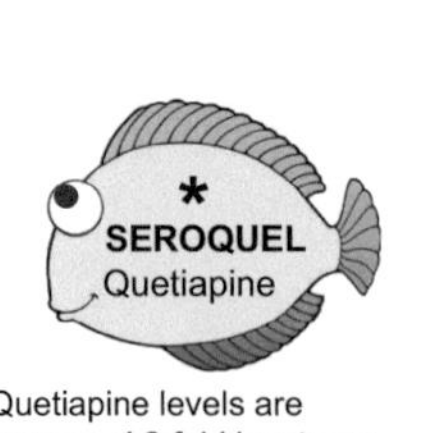

Lurasidone is metabolized exclusively by 3A4 and is contraindicated with potent 3A4 inhibitors or inducers.

Quetiapine levels are increased 6-fold by strong 3A4 inhibitors and decreased 6-fold by strong inducers.

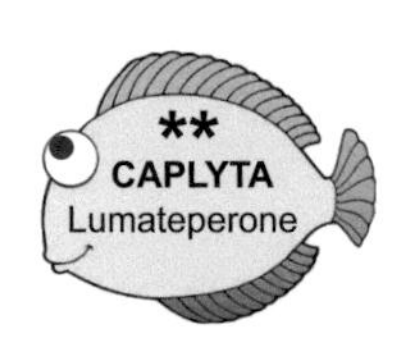

also 2D6

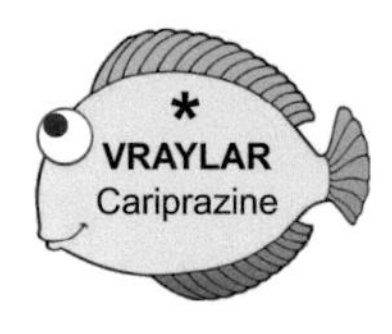

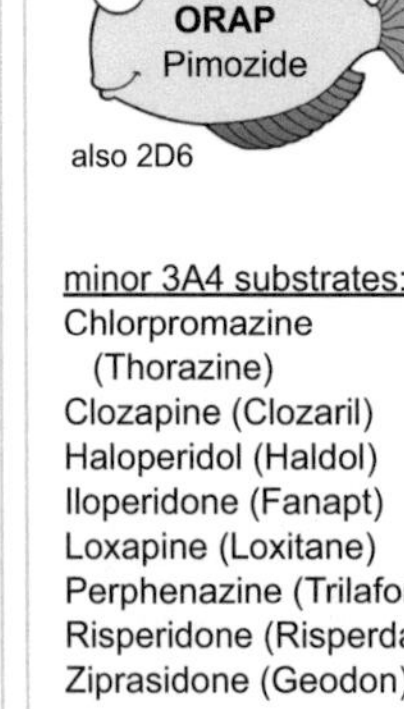
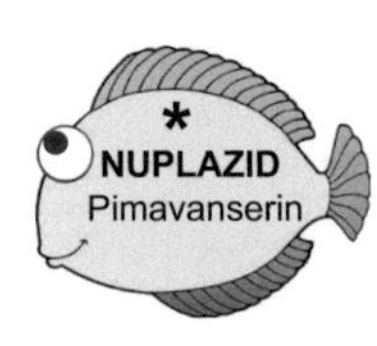

also 2D6

minor 3A4 substrates:
Chlorpromazine (Thorazine)
Clozapine (Clozaril)
Haloperidol (Haldol)
Iloperidone (Fanapt)
Loxapine (Loxitane)
Perphenazine (Trilafon)
Risperidone (Risperdal)
Ziprasidone (Geodon)

not:
Asenapine (Saphris) 1A2
Fluphenazine (Prolixin) 2D6
Molindone (Moban)
Olanzapine (Zyprexa) 1A2
Paliperidone (Invega)
Promethazine (Phenergan)
Thiothixene (Navane) 1A2
Trifluoperazine (Stelazine) 1A2

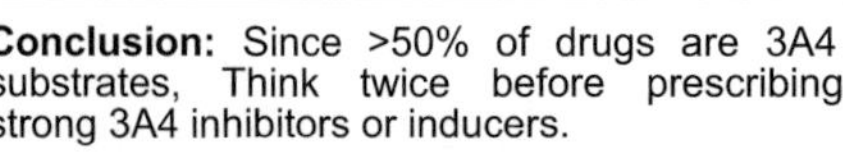

Conclusion: Since >50% of drugs are 3A4 substrates, Think twice before prescribing strong 3A4 inhibitors or inducers.

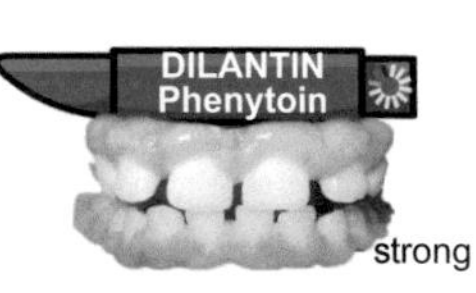

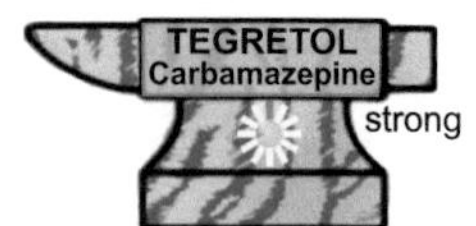

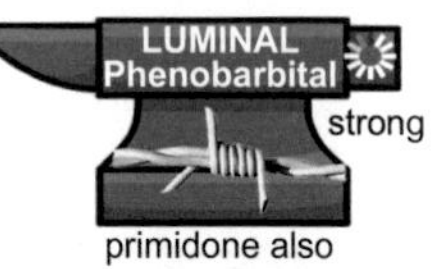

primidone also

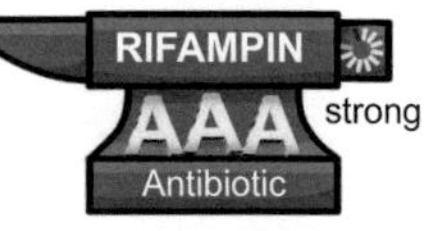

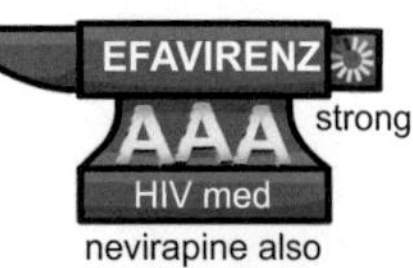

nevirapine also

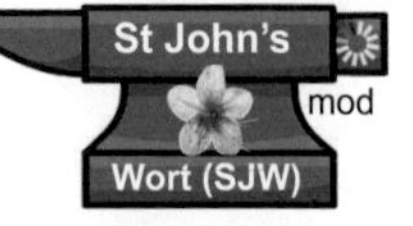

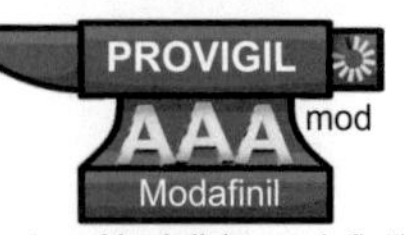

weaker: Nuvigil (armodafinil)

* Dosing adjustments defined

** Has contraindications related to kinetic interactions

UGT interactions

Phase II metabolism

18% of individuals are UGT1A4 ultrarapid metabolizers; 0% are poor metabolizers

There are two phases of drug metabolism. CYP enzymes are responsible for most phase I reactions, which make chemicals less fat-soluble (i.e., more water-soluble), usually by oxidation. Phase II reactions are usually by conjugation with glucuronic acid to render the chemical even more water-soluble. Chemicals conjugated with glucuronic acid are ready to be excreted in the urine or feces. The main phase II enzyme is UDP-glucuronosyltransferase (UGT), as in "U Got Tagged!" with glucuronic acid. The most relevant specific UGT enzyme for lamotrigine metabolism is UGT1A4.

Mood stabilizers metabolized by Phase II conjugation include valproic acid (VPA) and lamotrigine (Lamictal). UGT enzymes attach more strongly to VPA than to lamotrigine.

The presence of VPA slows the rate of Phase II metabolism of lamotrigine, causing lamotrigine blood levels to double.

There are several glucuronidation pathways involving several specific UGT enzymes. In this book, UGT activity and phase II metabolism are only visualized in the context of lamotrigine and the antipsychotic lumateperone (Caplyta)—both substrates of UGT1A4. Other UGT1A4 substrates (that could be depicted as sheep) include amitriptyline, doxepin, valproate, haloperidol, clozapine, olanzapine, and asenapine. GeneSight reports UGT**1A**4 and UGT**2B**15 (easy-to-recall sequence) metabolizer genotypes.

UGT2B15 is not visualized in this book. UGT2**B**15 substrates include the "LOT" **B**enzos—lorazepam, oxazepam and temazepam. The major UGT2B15 inHibitor is VPA. Nobody is a UGT2B15 ultrarapid or poor metabolizer, although some individuals are intermediate metabolizers.

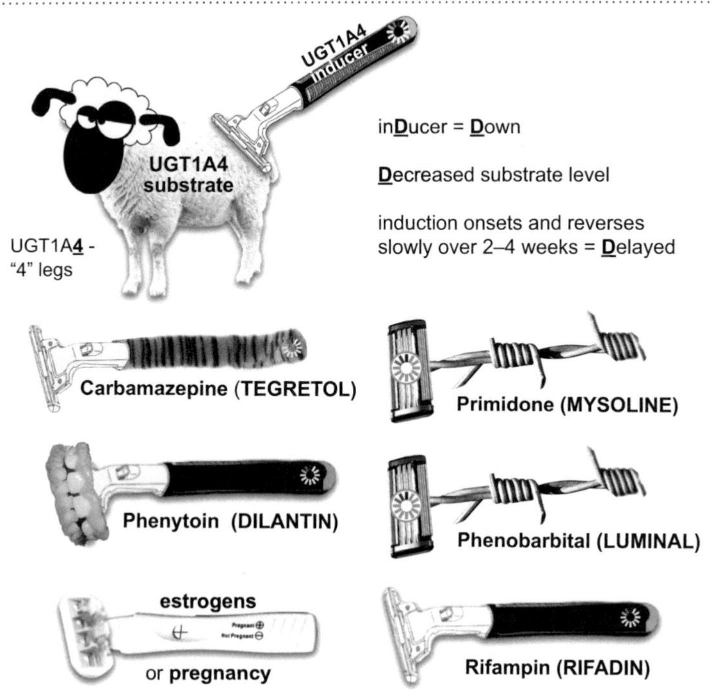

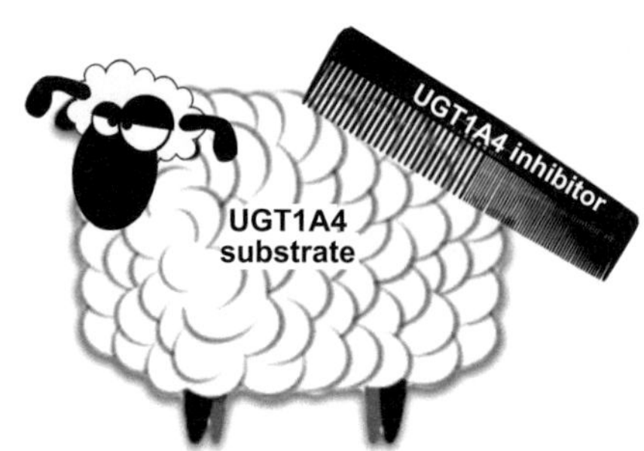

inHibitor = High

Increased substrate level

inHibition happens within Hours = Hurried

Inhibition reverses as soon as the inhibitor is cleared from the body (five half-lives of the inhibitor). In the case of VPA, 5 x 14 hours = about 3 days.

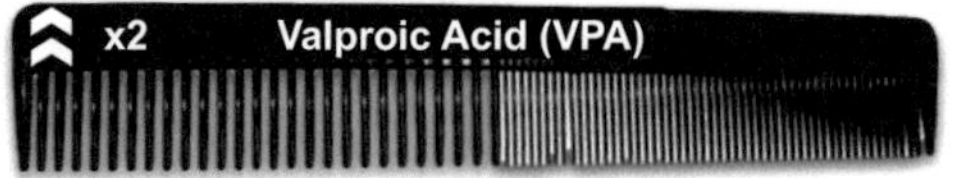

VPA doubles lamotrigine levels.

UGT1A4 substrates

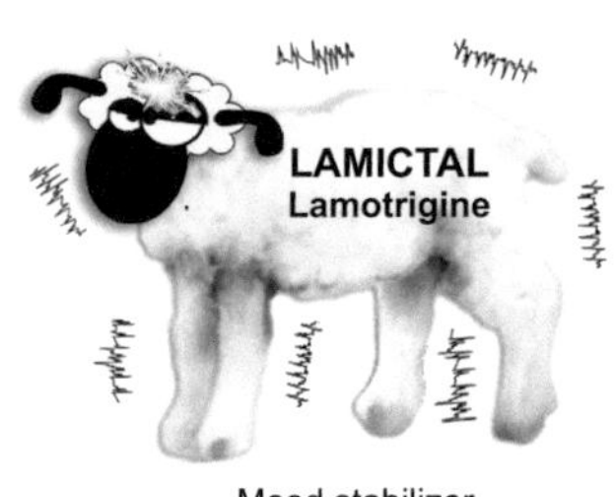

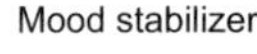
Mood stabilizer

Featured in *Cafer's Antipsychotics* book

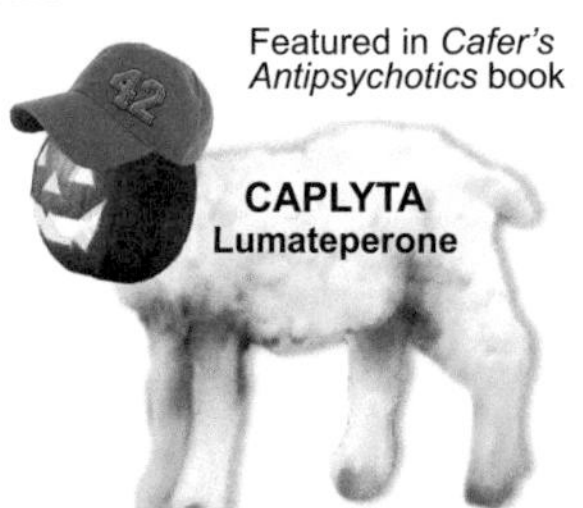

Antipsychotic

UGT1A4 ultrarapid metabolizers (UM)

Represented by a fast-shedding sheep, individuals who have a UGT1A4 ultrarapid metabolizer genotype clear UGT1A4 substrates quickly. These individuals are more likely to be non-responders to lamotrigine and lumateperone.

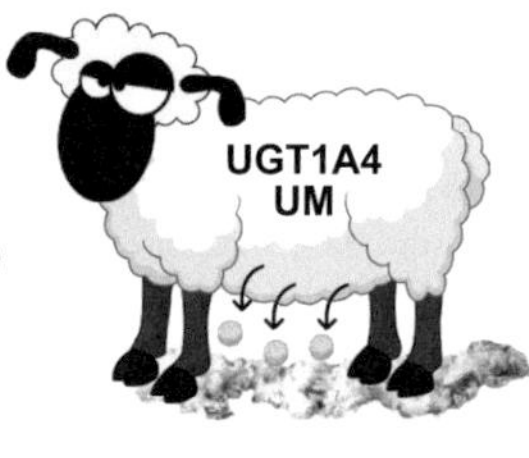

18% of population

Before lamotrigine became generically available, three Lamictal starter packs were available to address these interactions:

Starter pack	For those taking	Lamotrigine dose
Orange	No interacting medications	25 mg x 2 weeks, then 50 mg x 2 weeks, then 100 mg x 1 week. The usual maintenance dose starting on week 6 is 200 mg.
Blue	Valproate (Depakote)	Half strength. Maintenance dose is 100 mg QD.
Green	Carbamazepine (Tegretol) Phenytoin (Dilantin) Phenobarbital (Luminal) Primidone (Mysoline)	Double strength. Maintenance dose is 200 mg BID.

Lamotrigine and pregnancy: Lamotrigine is considered the safest anticonvulsant for pregnancy. It is non-teratogenic, other than a small risk of cleft palate.

Since **pregnancy can reduce lamotrigine levels by 50%**, it may be necessary to dose it higher during pregnancy and lower it upon childbirth. Compared with the early third trimester, postpartum lamotrigine serum levels increased an average of 172% (range 24–428%) within 5 weeks of giving birth (Clark et al, 2013).

At delivery, the mean umbilical cord lamotrigine level is ⅔ of the maternal level. In breastfed infants, the mean lamotrigine level in the child's blood is ⅓ of the maternal level. This is higher than expected with most drugs.

Conclusion: In management of bipolar disorder, lamotrigine can be combined with any mood stabilizer or antipsychotic. Lamictal plus lithium is a favorable pairing, as long as renal function is normal. The combination of lamotrigine and VPA may increase the risk of Stevens-Johnson syndrome. For patients on lamotrigine plus VPA or carbamazepine (CMZ), consider checking lamotrigine blood levels before discontinuation of VPA/CMZ and after lamotrigine dose is adjusted to account for reversal of inhibition/induction (page 7).

Non-participants

Medications that do not become significantly involved in kinetic interactions are depicted **"in a bubble"**.

Some of these medications are **"in a box"** (with a hole in it) to indicate that kinetic interactions exist, but usually do not need be taken into consideration when prescribing the medication.

Dynamic interactions still apply to bubbled/boxed medications.

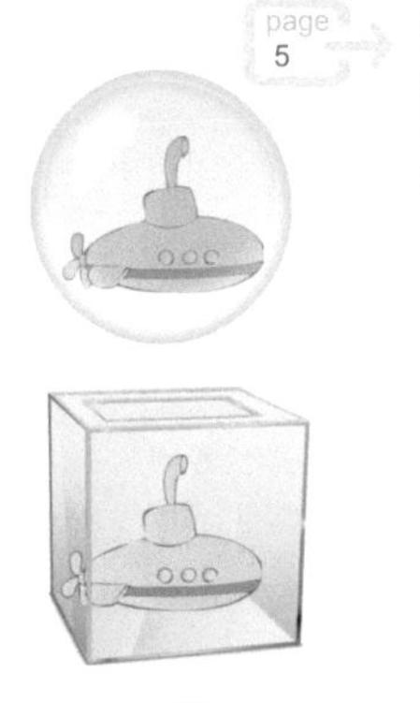

We will display medications "in a bubble" or "in a box" if they are not expected to serve as *clinically significant* substrates, inducers or inhibitors. There is a hole at the top of the boxes to indicate slight vulnerability to relevant kinetic interactions, but not to an extent prescribers need to worry about unless genetic testing reveals the patient to be a poor metabolizer for multiple CYP enzymes. In general, medications that are renally cleared have relatively few drug–drug interactions because their metabolism does not rely on hepatic enzymes.

For a substrate metabolized through multiple pathways, serum levels are not significantly affected by in**Hi**bition of a single CYP. For instance, over half of prescription drugs are 3A4 substrates, but they will probably not be depicted as fish (page 16) if they are multi-CYP substrates. Multi-CYP substrates are depicted in a box (not a bubble) because interactions do occur but are unlikely to matter much.

A multi-CYP substrate is more likely to be victimized by an in**D**ucer than by an in**H**ibitor. It is worthwhile to run an interaction check on a patient's medication list if they are taking a "shredder" in**D**ucer (page 7), even for the boxed medications.

A bubble/box certifies the medication is:

- ❖ No worse than a mild CYP inducer or inducer, and...
- ❖ Either a multi-CYP substrate or a substrate not metabolized by any CYP

A bubble does **not** imply that a medication does not participate in dynamic interactions, because almost all drugs do. Acamprosate (Campral) and N-acetylcysteine (NAC) are rare exceptions, depicted in a double bubble.

Cafer's Psychopharmacology contains over 270 monographs of medications with mascots designed to help you pair trade names with generic names, and to remember kinetic interactions. The mascots inside the bubbles/boxes are introduced in other books in this series.

Dynamic interactions:
Not applicable to every drug in class

"Bubbled" or "boxed" medications are unlikely to be involved in clinically significant kinetic interactions:

Antipsychotics

- ❖ EPS
- ❖ Sedation
- ❖ Weight gain
- ❖ Hyperglycemia
- ❖ QT prolongation
- ❖ Myelosuppression
- ❖ Anticholinergic
- ❖ Proconvulsant

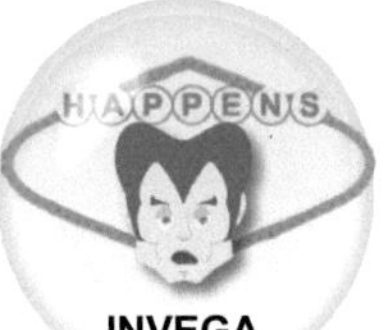

Paliperidone

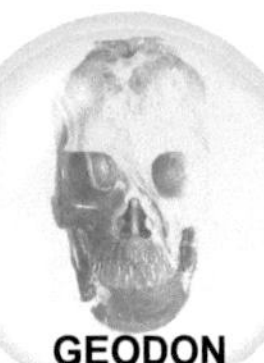

Ziprasidone

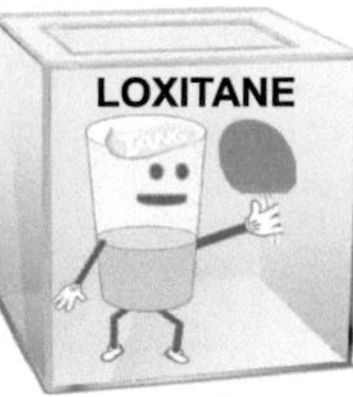

Loxapine

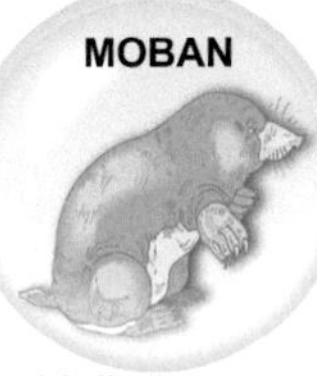

Molindone

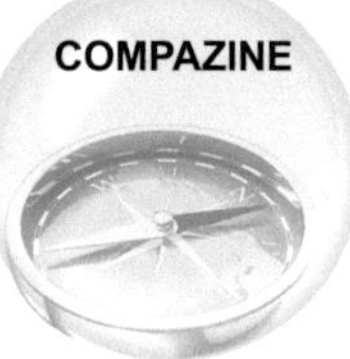

Prochlorperazine

Antidepressants

- ❖ Serotonergic
- ❖ QT prolongation
- ❖ Sedation (some)
- ❖ Weight gain
- ❖ Hyponatremia
- ❖ Antiplatelet
- ❖ Hypotensive (some)
- ❖ Hypertensive (others)

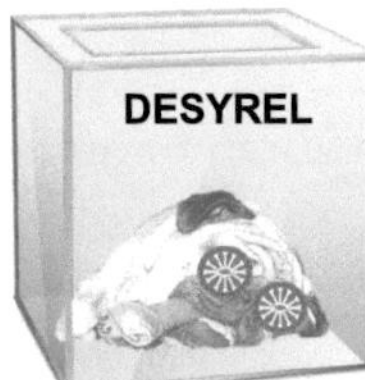

Trazodone

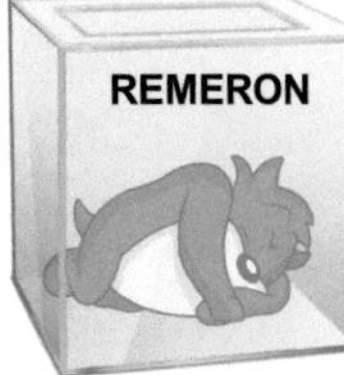

Mirtazapine

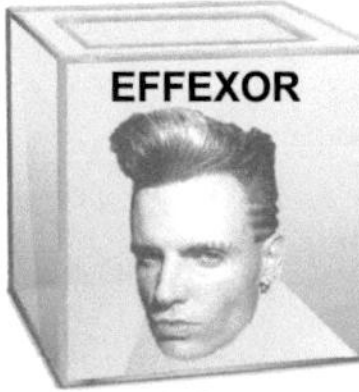

Venlafaxine

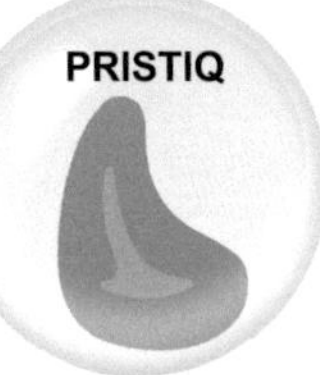

Desvenlafaxine

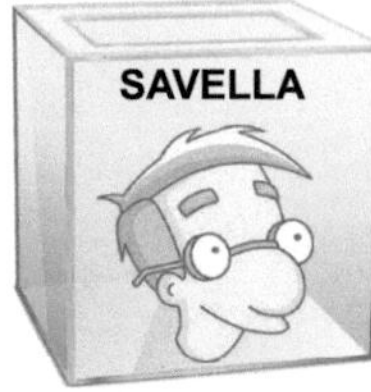

Milnacipran

Antiepileptics

- ❖ Sedation
- ❖ Stevens-Johnson Syndrome (page 28)
- ❖ Hyponatremia (page 33)
- ❖ Acidosis
- ❖ Myelosuppression

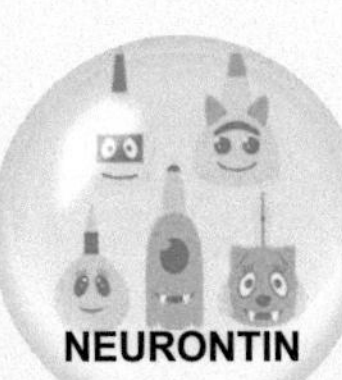

Gabapentin

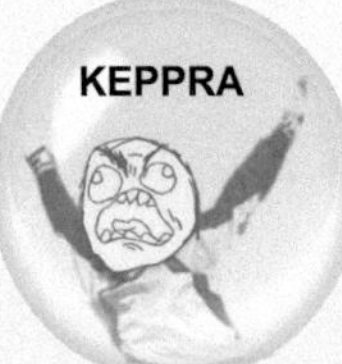

Levetiracetam

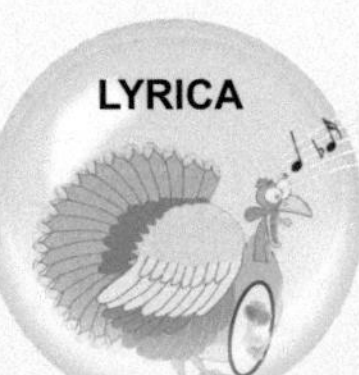

Pregabalin

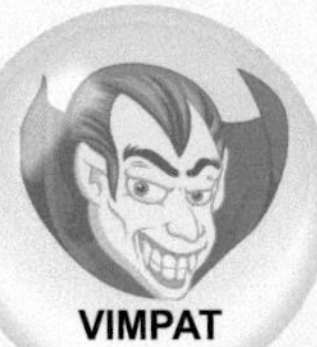

Lacosamide

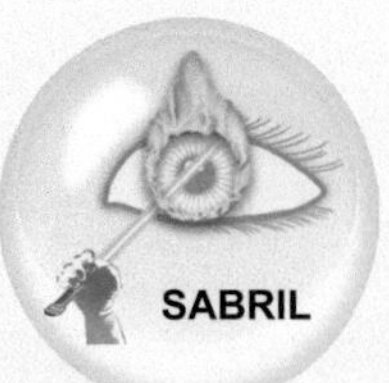

Vigabatrin

Sedatives

- ❖ Sedation
- ❖ Respiratory depression

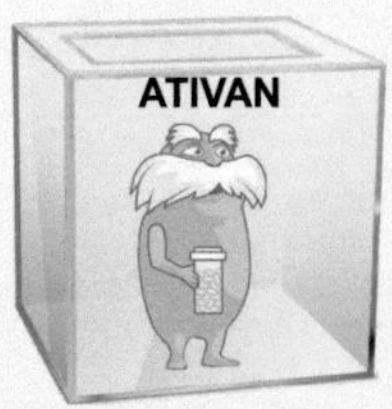

Lorazepam

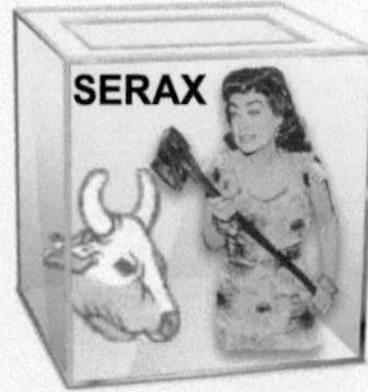

Oxazepam

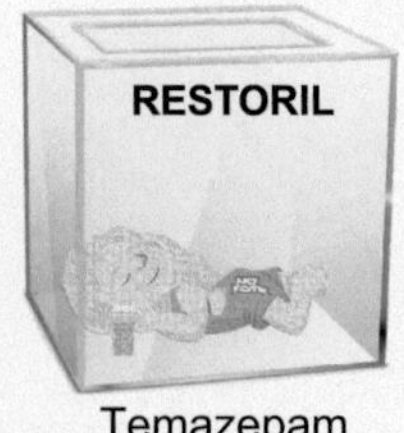

Temazepam

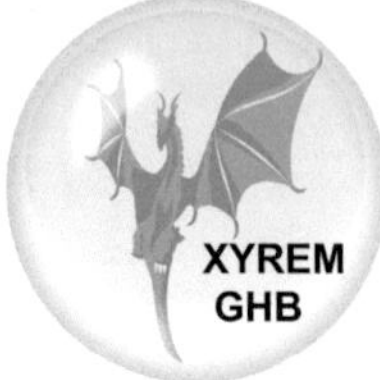

Sodium Oxybate

The 3 "LOT" benzos—No CYP interactions but levels may double due to UGT2B15 inHibition with VPA (Depakote)

Dynamic interactions:
Not applicable to every drug in class

"Bubbled" or "boxed" medications are unlikely to be involved in clinically significant <u>kinetic</u> interactions:

<u>Antihistamines</u>

- ❖ Anticholinergic
  - constipation
  - urinary retention
  - cognitive impairment
- ❖ Sedation

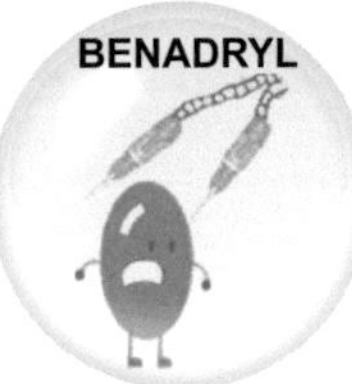

Diphenhydramine

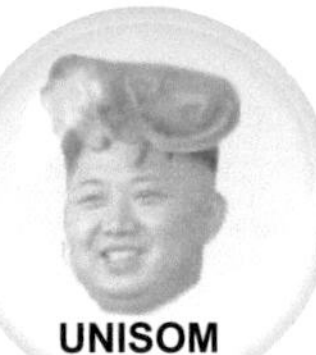

Doxylamine

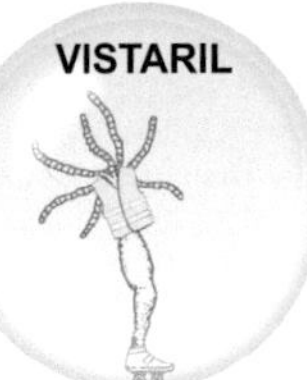

Hydroxyzine

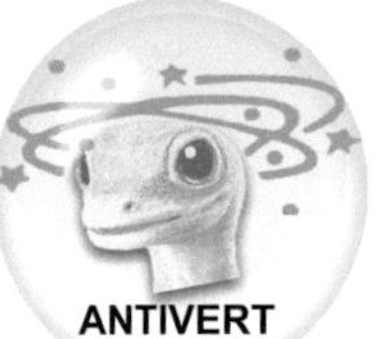

Meclizine

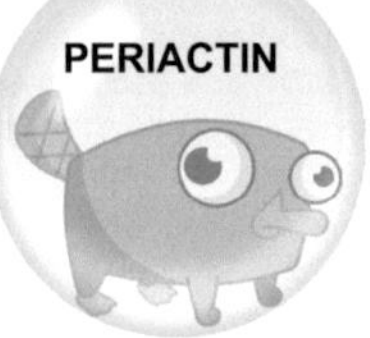

Cyproheptadine

<u>Anticholinergics</u>

- ❖ Anticholinergic
  - constipation
  - urinary retention
  - cognitive impairment
- ❖ Sedation

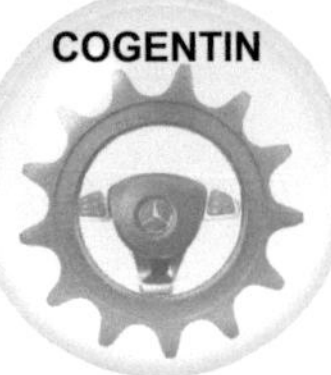

Benztropine

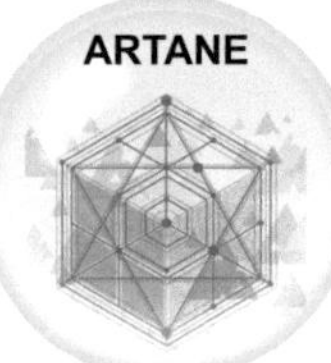

Trihexyphenidyl

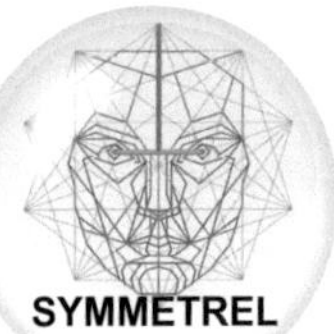

Amantadine

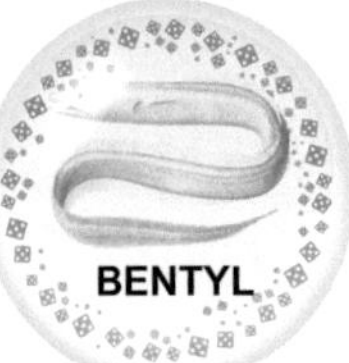

Dicyclomine

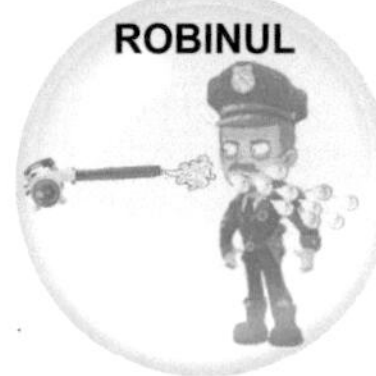

Glycopyrrolate

<u>Cognitive Enhancers</u>

- ❖ Cholinergic
- ❖ Proconvulsant

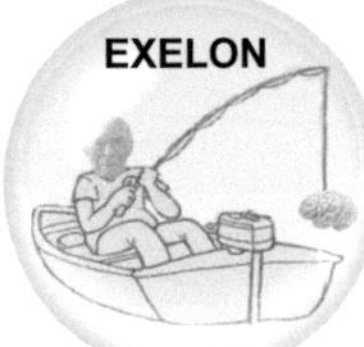

Rivastigmine

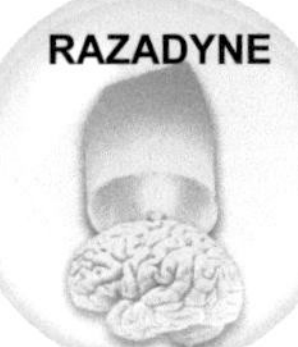

Galantamine

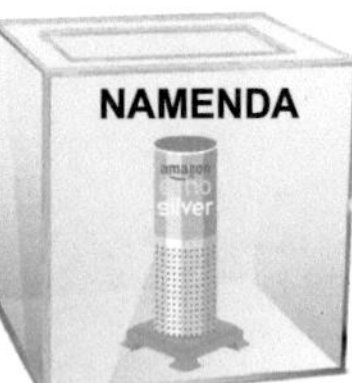

Memantine

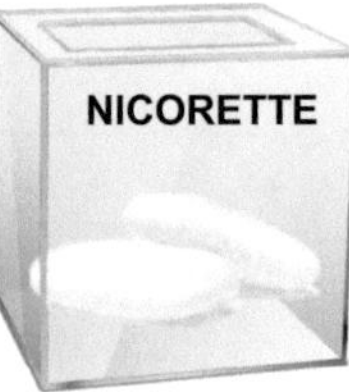

Nicotine

The hydrocarbons in smoked tobacco in**D**uce 1A2. Nicotine itself does not.

<u>Addiction Medicine</u>

For some, dynamic interactions are part of their mechanism of action, e.g., opioid antagonism by naltrexone and naloxone.

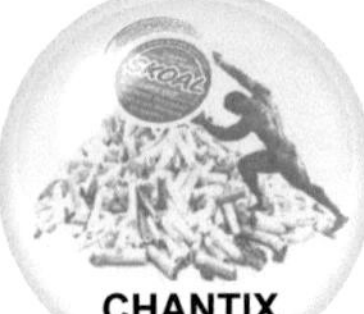

Varenicline

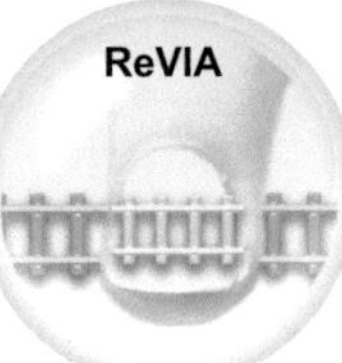

Naltrexone

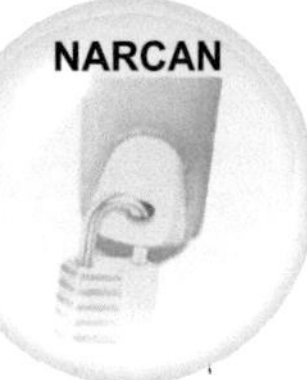

Naloxone

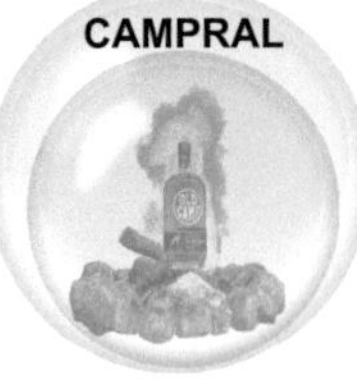

Acamprosate

Double bubble: Campral has no known kinetic or dynamic interactions.

<u>Antihypertensives</u>

- ❖ Hypotension
- ❖ Bradycardia
- ❖ Sedation
- ❖ Depression (some)

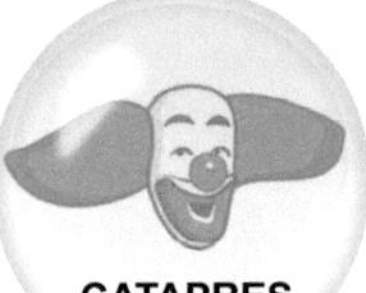

Clonidine

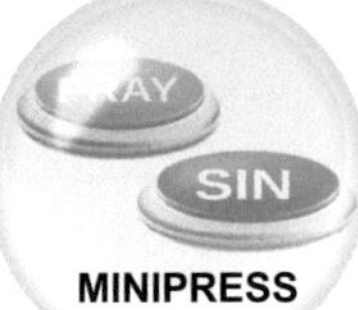

Prazosin

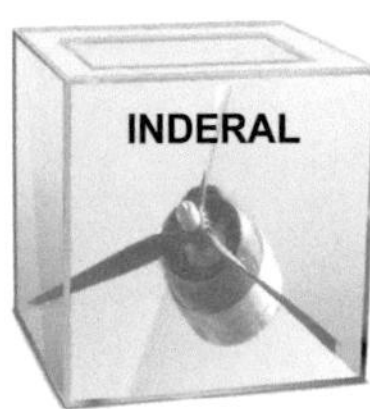

Propranolol

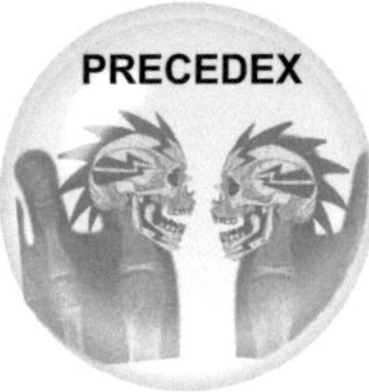

Dexmedetomidine

<u>Spasmolytics</u>

- ❖ Sedative
- ❖ Hypotensive
- ❖ Proconvulsant (some)

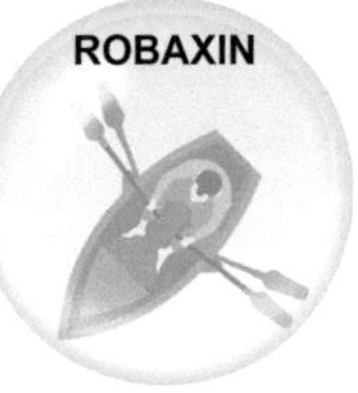

Methocarbamol

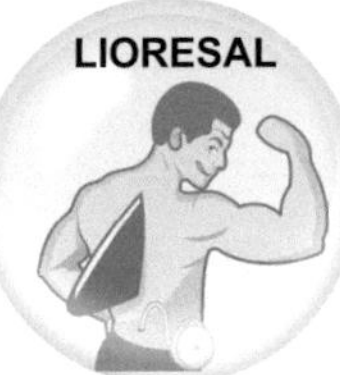

Baclofen

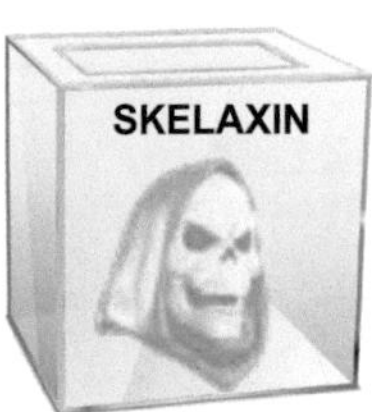

Metaxalone

<u>Stimulants</u>

- ❖ Proconvulsant
- ❖ Hypertensive
- ❖ Dopaminergic
- ❖ Noradrenergic

RITALIN
Methylphenidate

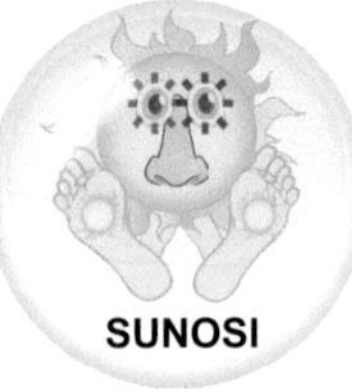

Solriamfetol

<u>Supplements</u>

Double bubble: NAC has no known kinetic or dynamic interactions.

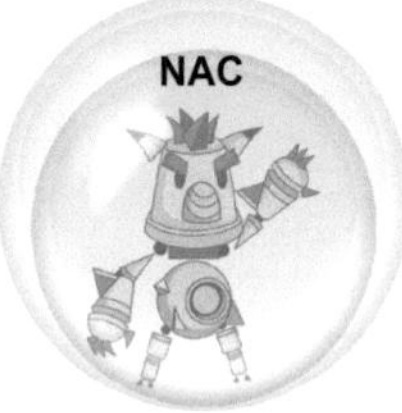

N-acetylcysteine

RELEVANT PHARMACOKINETIC INTERACTIONS, general overview

INDUCERS	INHIBITORS	SUBSTRATES
In**D**uction **D**ecreases substrates slowly, over 2 to 4 weeks (**D**elayed). With smoked tobacco, induction (1A2) starts in 3 days and reverses in about 1 week	In**H**ibition increases substrate levels (**H**igh), happening within **H**ours (**H**urried). Inhibition reverses as soon as the inhibitor is cleared from the body (five half-lives of the inhibitor)	"Victims" of inducers and inhibitors
1A2 inducers Ψ Tobacco/Cannabis (faster on/off) Ψ Carbamazepine Ψ Phenytoin	1A2 inhibitors Ψ **Fluvoxamine** Ciprofloxacin	1A2 substrates Ψ Asenapine Ψ **Clozapine** Ψ Duloxetine Ψ Olanzapine Ψ **Ramelteon** Ψ Thiothixene
2B6 inducers Ψ Carbamazepine Rifampin HIV MEDS	2B6 inhibitors Ψ Orphenadrine (Norflex)	2B6 substrates HIV MEDS CANCER MEDS Ψ Bupropion Ψ Ketamine Ψ Methadone Ψ Selegiline
2C9 inducers **Rifampin** Ψ St John's Wort	2C9 inhibitors **Fluconazole**	2C9 substrates Ψ Valproate (VPA)
2C19 inducers Ψ Phenobarbital Rifampin Apalutamide ***Ultrarapid metabolizers (10%)***	2C19 inhibitors Ψ **Cannabidiol** (CBD) **Fluconazole** Ψ Fluoxetine Ψ Fluvoxamine ***Poor metabolizers (5%)***	2C19 substrates Ψ Citalopram Ψ Diazepam Ψ Escitalopram Ψ Phenobarbital Ψ Phenytoin Ψ Sertraline Ψ Methadone Warfarin
2D6 inducers None ***Ultrarapid metabolizers (5%)***	2D6 inhibitors Ψ **Bupropion** Ψ Duloxetine Ψ **Fluoxetine** Ψ **Paroxetine** **Quinidine** ***Poor metabolizers (10%)***	2D6 substrates Ψ Tricyclics (TCAs) Ψ Aripiprazole Ψ Atomoxetine Ψ Brexpiprazole Ψ Bupropion-OH Ψ Codeine *PRODRUG* Ψ Deutetrabenazine Ψ Dextromethorphan Ψ Duloxetine Ψ Haloperidol Ψ Iloperidone Ψ **Perphenazine** Ψ **Pimozide** Ψ Risperidone Tamoxifen *PRODRUG* Ψ Tetrabenazine Ψ **Thioridazine** Ψ Tramadol *PRODRUG* Ψ Vortioxetine
3A4 inducers Ψ **Carbamazepine** Ψ Modafinil Ψ **Phenobarbital** Ψ **Phenytoin** **Rifampin** Ψ St John's Wort	3A4 inhibitors Protease Inhibitors (HIV) Clarithromycin Diltiazem Grapefruit juice **Ketoconazole** **Itraconazole** Ψ **Nefazodone** Verapamil	3A4 substrates Immunosuppressants Progestins Ψ Alprazolam Ψ Aripiprazole Ψ Brexpiprazole Ψ Buprenorphine Ψ **Buspirone** Ψ Carbamazepine Ψ Cariprazine Ψ Chlordiazepoxide Ψ Clonazepam Ψ **Flibanserin** Ψ Lemborexant Ψ **Lumateperone** Ψ **Lurasidone** Ψ Pimavanserin Ψ Pimozide Ψ **Quetiapine** Sildenafil **Simvastatin** Ψ Suvorexant Tadalafil Ψ Valbenazine Ψ **Vilazodone**
UGT inducers Ψ Carbamazepine Estrogens Ψ Phenobarbital Ψ Phenytoin Rifampin	UGT inhibitors Ψ **Valproate (VPA)**	UGT substrates Ψ **Lamotrigine** Ψ **Lumateperone**

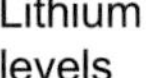

Lithium levels

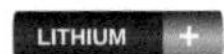

Decreased by:
- Acetazolamide
- Ψ Caffeine
- Mannitol
- Theophylline
- Ψ Topiramate
- Ψ Zonisamide

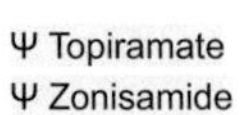

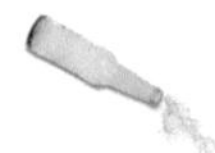

Increased by:

Thiazides:
- HCTZ
- Chlorthalidone

NSAIDS:
- Celebrex
- Ibuprofen
- Indomethacin
- Naproxen
- Diclofenac

ACE Inhibitors "-prils"

ARBs "-sartans"

Antimicrobials:
- Tetracyclines
- Metronidazole

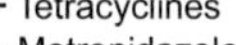

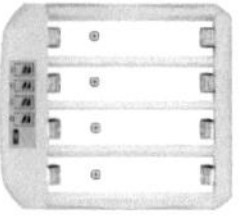

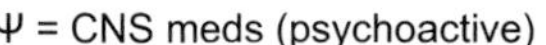

Ψ = CNS meds (psychoactive)

Pharmacokinetic Drug-Drug Interactions

INDUCERS

InDuction decreases (Down) substrates slowly, over 2 to 4 weeks* (Delayed).

Inducer	CYP
Ψ Armodafinil	(3A4) weak
Apalutamide (prostate cancer)	2C19, 3A4 & (2C9)
Ψ Cannabis	1A2 fast
Chargrilled meat	1A2
Ψ Carbamazepine (Tegretol)	3A4, 2B6 & (1A2)
Efavirenz (HIV)	3A4, 2B6
Enzalutamide (prostate cancer)	3A4, 2C9 & 2C19
Estradiol	UGT
Ψ Modafinil	3A4
Nevirapine	2B6 (3A4)
Ψ Phenobarbital (Luminal)	3A4 (1A2), (2B6, 2C9) & UGT
Ψ Phenytoin (Dilantin)	3A4 (1A2), (2B6), UGT
Ψ Primidone (Mysoline) metab to phenobarb	3A4 (1A2), (2B6, 2C9) & UGT
Rifampin (Rifadin)	2C19, 3A4, 2B6, 2C9 (1A2) & UGT
Ritonavir (HIV)	2B6 (2C19) (1A2, 2C9)
Ψ St John's Wort	1A2, 2C9 & 3A4
Ψ Tobacco	1A2 fast
Ψ Topiramate ≥200 mg	(3A4)

inDuction reverses gradually over a few weeks* after the inducer is discontinued.

*With smoking (tobacco or cannabis), induction is faster (a few days).

INHIBITORS

InHibition increases substrate levels (High). Inhibition happens within Hours (Hurried).

Inhibitor	CYP
Amiodarone	(2C9, 2D6, 3A4)
Ψ Asenapine	(2D6) weak
Ψ Bupropion	2D6
Ψ Cannabidiol	2C19, UGT
Cimetidine	(multi) weak
Ciprofloxacin	1A2, (3A4)
Clarithromycin	3A4
Clopidogrel	(2B6)
Darunavir (HIV)	3A4, (2D6)
Diltiazem	3A4, (2D6)
Ψ Duloxetine	2D6
Efavirenz (HIV)	2C9, 2C19
Erythromycin	3A4
Esomeprazole	(2C19) weak
Fluconazole	2C9, 2C19, 3A4
Ψ Fluoxetine	2D6, 2C19
Ψ Fluvoxamine (Luvox)	1A2, 2C19, & (3A4, 2C9)
Grapefruit juice	3A4
Isoniazid	(3A4) weak
Indinavir	3A4
Itraconazole	3A4
Ketoconazole	3A4, (2C19)
Ψ Methadone	(2D6) weak
Ψ Modafinil	(2C19) weak
Nelfinavir	3A4
Omeprazole	2C19
Ψ Nefazodone	3A4
Ψ Orphenadrine	2B6
Ψ Paroxetine	2D6
Quinidine	2D6, (3A4)
Ritonavir	3A4 Black Box
Ψ Sertraline ≥150mg	(2D6)
Terbinafine	2D6
Ψ Thioridazine	2D6
Ψ Valproate (VPA)	UGT-1A & -2B
Voriconazole	3A4,2C19,(2C9)
Verapamil	3A4, (1A2)

InHibition is reversed as soon as the inhibitor is cleared, which will be about 5 half-lives after it is discontinued.

UGT & UGT-1A refer to UGT1A4. UGT-2B refers to UGT2B15.

( ) = weak inducer/inhibitor; less susceptible substrate

Ψ = CNS medication (psychoactive)

SUBSTRATES

"Victims" of inducers and inhibitors

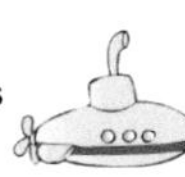

In general, substrates that are metabolized through only one pathway are more vulnerable to drug interactions. For drugs metabolized by multiple CYPs, strong inDuction of a single CYP is likely to reduce substrate levels, but inHibition of one CYP is unlikely to significantly increase substrate levels.

Substrate	CYP
Atazanavir (HIV)	3A4
Ψ Alprazolam	3A4
Ψ Amitriptyline	2D6, 2C19
Amlodipine	3A4
Ψ Amoxapine	2D6
Ψ Amphetamine salts	(2D6)
Ψ Aripiprazole	2D6, 3A4
Ψ Armodafinil	3A4
Ψ Asenapine	(1A2)
Ψ Atomoxetine	2D6, (2C19)
Atorvastatin	3A4
Avanafil	3A4
Ψ Brexpiprazole	2D6, 3A4
Ψ Buprenorphine	3A4
Ψ Bupropion	2B6; 2D6 (OH-)
Ψ Buspirone	3A4, (2D6)
Ψ Caffeine	1A2 (etc)
Ψ Carbamazepine	3A4
Ψ Cariprazine	3A4, (2D6)
Ψ Carisoprodol	2C19
Carvedilol	2D6 (etc)
Celecoxib	2C9, (3A4)
Ψ Chlordiazepoxide	3A4
Ψ Chlorpromazine	2D6, (1A2,3A4)
Ψ Citalopram	2C19,3A4(2D6)
Clarithromycin	3A4
Ψ Clomipramine	2D6, 2C19, 1A2
Ψ Clonazepam	3A4
Clopidogrel	2C19, (3A4)
Ψ Clozapine	1A2 (2D6, etc)
Ψ Codeine *2D6 prodrug	*2D6, (3A4)
Ψ Cyclobenzaprine	1A2, (2D6, 3A4)
Cyclophosphamide	2B6, 2C19
Cyclosporine	3A4 (etc)
Ψ Desipramine	2D6, (1A2)
Ψ Deutetrabenazine	2D6
Ψ Dextromethorphan	2D6 (etc)
Ψ Diazepam	2C19, 3A4
Diclofenac	multi
Diltiazem	3A4 (2C19,3A4)
Ψ Doxepin	2D6, 2C19 (etc)
Ψ Donepezil	(2D6, 3A4)
Ψ Duloxetine	2D6, 1A2
Efavirenz (HIV)	2B6, 3A4
Ψ Escitalopram	2C19,3A4(2D6)
Esomeprazole	2C19, (3A4)
Estradiol	1A2, 2C9, 3A4
Ψ Eszopiclone	3A4
Ψ Fentanyl 3A4 Black Box	3A4 (etc)
Flecainide	2D6, 1A2
Ψ Flibanserin 3A4 Black Box	3A4, 2C9, 2C19
Ψ Fluoxetine	2D6, 2C9 (etc)
Ψ Fluphenazine	2D6
Ψ Flurazepam	3A4
Fluvastatin	2C9 (2B6, 3A4)
Ψ Fluvoxamine	2D6, 1A2
Ψ Galantamine	(2D6, 3A4)
Glimepiride	2C9
Glipizide	2C9
Glyburide	2C9
Ψ Guanfacine	3A4
Ψ Haloperidol	2D6, 3A4, (1A2)
Ψ Hydrocodone Black Box	3A4
Ifosfamide	2B6 (& others)
Ψ Iloperidone	2D6, (3A4)
Ψ Imipramine	2D6, 2C19 (etc)
Ψ Ketamine	2B6, 2C9, 3A4
Ψ Lamotrigine	UGT
Lansoprazole	2C19, 3A4
Ψ Lemborexant	3A4
Ψ Levomilnacipran	3A4, (2D6)
Ψ Lorazepam	UGT-2B (VPA)
Losartan	2C9, 3A4
Ψ Loxapine	(1A2, 2D6,3A4)
Ψ Lumateperone	3A4, UGT-1A
Ψ Lurasidone *contraind*	3A4
Medroxyprogesterone	3A4
Meloxicam	2C9, (3A4)
Ψ Meperidine Black Box	3A4
Ψ Methadone	3A4, 2B6, (etc)
Ψ Methamphetamine	2D6
Metoprolol	2D6, (2C19)
Mexiletine	1A2, 2D6
Ψ Midazolam	3A4, (2B6)
Ψ Mirtazapine	2D6, 3A4, 1A2
Ψ Modafinil	3A4 (2D6)
Nevirapine	3A4 (2B6, 2D6)
Ψ Nefazodone	3A4; 2D6 mCPP
Nifedipine	3A4, (2D6)
Norethindrone	3A4
Ψ Nortriptyline	2D6 (etc)
Ψ Olanzapine	1A2; (2D6)
Omeprazole	2C19 (etc)
Ψ Oxazepam	UGT-2B (VPA)
Ψ Oxycodone	3A4, (2D6)
Pantoprazole	2C19,(2D6, 3A4)
Ψ Paroxetine	2D6
Ψ Perphenazine	2D6 (etc)
Ψ Phenobarbital	2C19,(2C9)
Ψ Phenytoin	2C9, 2C19,(3A4)
Ψ Pimavanserin	3A4
Ψ Pimozide	2D6, 3A4 (1A2)
Piroxicam	2C9
Ψ Promethazine	(2B6, 2D6)
Propafenone	2D6, (1A2, 3A4)
Ψ Propofol	2B6 (etc)
Ψ Propranolol	2D6, 1A2,(2C19)
Ψ Protriptyline	2D6
Ψ Quetiapine	3A4, (2D6)
Ψ Ramelteon	1A2 (3A4,2C19)
Ψ Risperidone	2D6, (3A4)
Ψ Selegiline	2B6 (etc)
Ψ Sertraline	2C19 (2B6,2D6)
Sildenafil	3A4, (etc)
Simvastatin	3A4
Ψ Suvorexant	3A4
Tacrolimus	3A4
Tadalafil	3A4
Tamoxifen *2D6 prodrug	*2D6, 3A4, 2C9
Ψ Tasimelteon	1A2, 3A4
Ψ Temazepam	UGT-2B (VPA)
Ψ Tetrabenazine	2D6
Theophylline	1A2, (3A4)
Ψ Thioridazine	2D6, (2C19)
Ψ Thiothixene	1A2
Ψ Tiagabine	3A4
Ψ Tizanidine	1A2
Tolbutamide	2C9, (2C19)
Ψ Tramadol *2D6 prodrug*	3A4,(2D6*; 2B6)
Ψ Trazodone	3A4 (2D6 mCPP)
Ψ Triazolam	3A4
Ψ Trifluoperazine	1A2
Ψ Trimipramine	2D6, 2C19, 3A4
Ψ Valproate (VPA)	(multi); Aspirin*
Ψ Valbenazine	3A4 (2D6)
Vardenafil	3A4
Ψ Venlafaxine	2D6, 3A4,(2C19)
Ψ Vilazodone	3A4,(2C19,2D6)
Vincristine	3A4
Voriconazole	2C9, 2C19, 3A4
Ψ Vortioxetine	2D6, 3A4, etc
Warfarin	2C9, 2C19,(3A4)
Ψ Zaleplon	(3A4)
Ψ Zolpidem	3A4 (etc)

Lithium levels

LITHIUM

Decreased by:

- Acetazolamide
- Ψ Caffeine
- Mannitol
- Theophylline
- Ψ Topiramate
- Ψ Zonisamide (weak)

Increased by:

- Benazepril
- Celecoxib
- Chlorthalidone
- Diclofenac
- Doxycycline
- Enalapril
- Etodolac
- HCTZ
- Ibuprofen
- Indomethacin
- Irbesartan Lisinopril
- Tetracycline
- Losartan
- Metronidazole
- Minocycline
- Naproxen
- Olmesartan
- Ramipril
- Valsartan

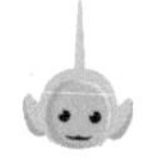

With high-dose aspirin, Depakote (VPA) will be stronger than suggested by total VPA level because aspirin (highly protein-bound) bumps VPA off of albumin (page 29).

Medication Monographs

#40 most prescribed US
1993
$4–$250

Chemical structure

Generic Name (TRADE NAME)

[pronunciation]

mnemonic phrase

❖ Class of medication
❖ Mechanism of action

100
<u>200</u>
400
mg

Year the drug was introduced to the U.S. market

Monographs focus on the unique aspects of the individual drug, to be taken in context of the medication class. Most of the medications in this book are psychotropic, i.e., capable of affecting the mind, emotions and behavior.

Price range for a month's supply of the generic (if available) version of the drug. The price is generally applicable to the most common prescription, which would be #30 for drugs usually dosed QD, #60 for those dosed BID, and #90 for those usually dosed TID. The applicable milligram strength is the number underlined in the upper righthand corner. The bottom dollar value is the lowest GoodRx price, available with a coupon at select pharmacies. The high dollar value is the average retail price in mid-late 2019. The wide price range from pharmacy to pharmacy shows the importance of checking a source like GoodRx prior to filling a script for cash.

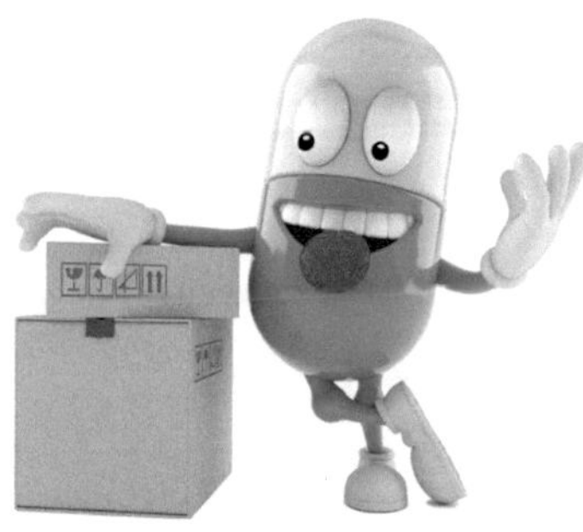

Each monograph features a mascot designed to pair the drug's generic name with the most common U.S. trade name.

A representative pill of the underlined strength, either a branded or generic version. The main purpose is to show whether we're talking capsules or tablets. For tablets, we try to show the side with score lines. If no score lines are shown, assume that the pill is not intended to be split. For any splittable psychotropic medication, giving a half dose for the first two days is a good idea.

Dosing: When provided, dosing recommendations are applicable to healthy adults. Refer to other sources for pediatric recommendations. Older adults should generally be given lower doses. Doses may need to be modified when considering kinetic/dynamic interactions and renal/hepatic insufficiency.

Boxes like this contain contextual information about the drug.

A link to a page with relevant content looks like this:

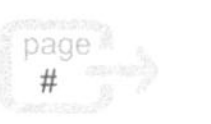

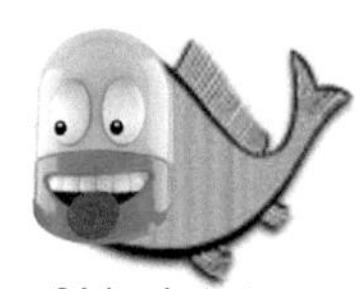

3A4 substrate

The box with rounded corners contains a visual hybrid of the mascot and CYP interaction mnemonic(s). Over half of prescription drugs are metabolized by 3A4, so there are plenty of fish.

Recurring Visuals

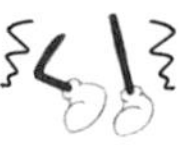

Dopaminergic medication for Restless Legs Syndrome (RLS)

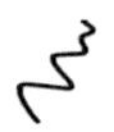

Medication for Parkinsonian tremor

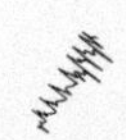

Antiepileptic drug (AED)

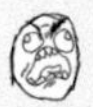

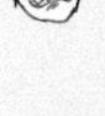

Medication that may cause agitation (various angry faces)

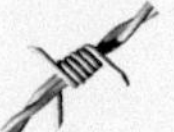

Barbiturate

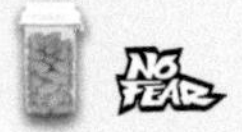

Benzodiazepine

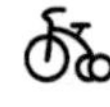

Tricyclic antidepressant (TCA)

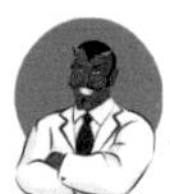

Antipsychotic (various spooky characters)

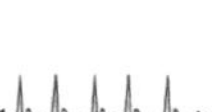

QT interval prolonging medication

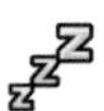

Non-benzodiazepine (Z-drug)

Antidepressant (rain cloud)

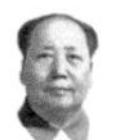

MAOI Inhibitor (Chairman MAO)

Anticholinergic with CNS effects (Mad as a hatter)

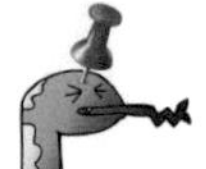

Antihistamine (push pin) – "anti-hiss-tamine"

Opioid (pinpoint pupils)

Opioid antagonist (dilated pupils)

Medication with stimulant properties/ wakefulness promoting agent

Antihypertensive/sympatholytic
- high pressure spray representing blood pressure

Amphetamine (Adderall, etc)

Methylphenidates (Ritalin, etc)
- Scantron sheet on "Math final date"

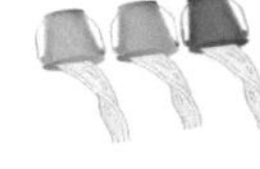

Cholinergic medication
- "SLUDGE buckets"

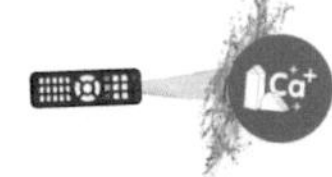

Calcium channel blocker

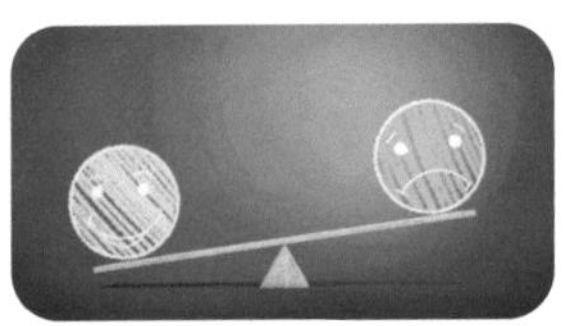

Mood Stabilizers

Mood stabilizers are used to treat bipolar disorder (type I and II). They can also be used off-label for mood swings characteristic of borderline personality disorder, preferably as an adjunct to Dialectical Behavior Therapy (DBT). With the exception of lithium, all mood stabilizers are antiepileptic drugs (AEDs). When stopping any AED, it is important to taper gradually. Abrupt discontinuation of an AED may cause a seizure, even with individuals without epilepsy.

Mood Stabilizer/monthly cost		Blood levels	Recommended lab work	Comments
Lithium Lithium IR (ESKALITH) Lithium ER (LITHOBID) Lithium Citrate Syrup	 $5 $20 $100	0.6–1.0 for maintenance 1.0–1.4 for acute mania	Lithium level TSH (hypothyroidism) CMP (renal insufficiency) EKG if cardiac disease Pregnancy test (Ebstein's anomaly)	Most effective medication for prevention of mania recurrence and lowering risk of suicide; Narrow therapeutic index; Risk of renal damage; Neuroprotective
Valproate Divalproex DR (DEPAKOTE) Divalproex ER (DEPAKOTE ER) Valproic Acid (DEPAKENE) syrup	 $15 $40 $25	50–100 for maintenance 80–120 for acute mania	Valproic acid (VPA) level CMP (liver) CBC (thrombocytopenia) Ammonia if suspicion of encephalopathy Pregnancy test (low IQ, neural tube)	Risk of hepatotoxicity; Significant tremor is possible (reversible)
Lamotrigine (LAMICTAL) Lamotrigine ER (LAMICTAL XR)	$10 $50	Not required (2–20)	None	Few side effects or health risks; Must titrate slowly to avoid SJS, making it useless for acute mania.
Carbamazepine (TEGRETOL) Carbamazepine XR (CARBATROL)	$40 $50	4–12 for seizure disorder undefined for bipolar disorder	Carbamazepine level (optional) CBC (anemia, neutropenia) CMP (sodium, liver) HLA-B*1502 for Asians (SJS) Pregnancy test (neural tube defects)	"Shredder" in**D**ucer of several CYP enzymes, **D**ecreasing levels of numerous medications; Blood levels required for treatment of epilepsy but not for bipolar maintenance.
Oxcarbazepine (TRILEPTAL)	$25	Not required (15–35)	Metabolic panel (low sodium) HLA-B*1502 for Asians (SJS)	Off-label for bipolar; Risk of hyponatremia

SJS = Stevens-Johnson Syndrome

Antiepileptics with (possible) weak mood stabilizing properties

Clinical guidelines generally consider these two medications to be non-mood stabilizing antiepileptics. However, some psychiatrists regard them as adjunctive stabilizers for bipolar disorder. At worst they are unlikely to destabilize mood, which is something that cannot be said of all antiepileptics.

Antiepileptic/monthly cost		Levels needed	Recommended lab work	Comments
Gabapentin (NEURONTIN)	$10	No	None	Off-label for anxiety, neuropathic pain, borderline personality, alcoholism, PTSD nightmares
Topiramate (TOPAMAX)	$10	No	CMP looking for low bicarbonate (CO_2) which indicates acidosis; Pregnancy test (hypospadias, oral clefts)	Causes cognitive impairment ≥ 200 mg; Off-label for weight loss

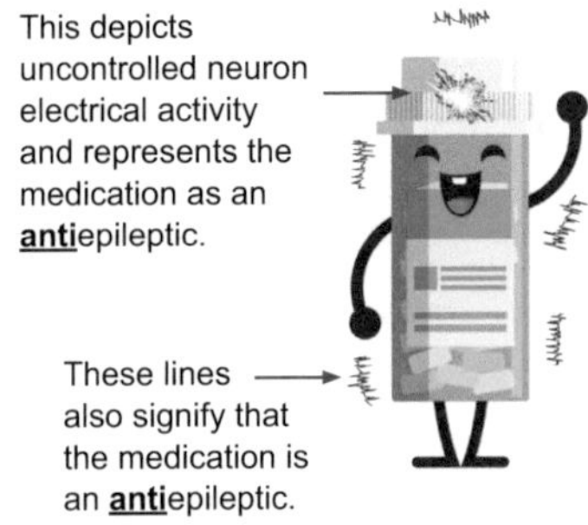

Antipsychotics are not considered mood stabilizers, but are used for similar purposes, often in combination with a stabilizer. Antipsychotics work faster than stabilizers to relieve acute mania. For acute mania, it is best to hospitalize the patient and use a stabilizer + antipsychotic + benzodiazepine. To minimize sedatives while treating mania, consider blue-light blocking glasses (as described on page 48) for experimental "virtual darkness therapy".

The benzo can be tapered off (or made PRN) while mania is resolving, and it may be possible to taper the antipsychotic within a few months. Keep the stabilizer on board to prevent recurrence of mania or replace it with lamotrigine (Lamictal) for maintenance. Lamotrigine is safer, has fewer side effects, and is effective for prevention of manic and depressive episodes. Antidepressants may be useful for bipolar depression in the short term but may destabilize mood when used long term for individuals with bipolar disorder.

Other than lithium, all mood stabilizers are AEDs, but not all AEDs are stabilizers. Bipolar patients on a non-stabilizing antiepileptic should, if possible, be switched to valproate, lamotrigine, carbamazepine, or oxcarbazepine (in collaboration with the neurologist).

The following medication monographs include a mechanism of action in the upper right-hand corner. Realize, however, the usual AED has several mechanisms of unclear significance. In general, AEDs enhance GABA activity and/or decrease glutamate activity. GABA is the brain's principal inhibitory neurotransmitter, while glutamate is the principal excitatory neurotransmitter. Several AEDs block voltage-gated sodium and/or voltage-gated calcium channels of presynaptic neurons.

#222
1970

LITHIUM

Lithium carbonate

Lithium citrate

Lithium orotate

- ❖ Mood stabilizer
- ❖ Neuroprotectant

FDA-approved for:

- ❖ Acute mania
- ❖ Bipolar disorder (maintenance)

Used off-label for:

- ❖ Depression
- ❖ Suicidal ideation
- ❖ Dementia
- ❖ Alcoholism
- ❖ Agitation
- ❖ Headaches
- ❖ Neutropenia
- ❖ SIADH
- ❖ Longevity

Lithium is the gold standard treatment for bipolar disorder. It is superior to all medications at preventing suicide, reducing risk 5-fold for individuals with recurrent unipolar depression and 6-fold for those with bipolar disorder (Tondo et al, 2016). It works by several mechanisms that are not entirely understood.

Lithium is an element on the periodic table, classified as an alkali metal. Its atomic number is 3, making it the 3rd lightest element. Lithium was one of the first three elements in existence with the big bang (along with helium and hydrogen) over 13 billion years ago.

Lithium citrate was added to 7-Up (originally known as Bib-Label Lithiated Lemon-Lime Soda) from 1929–1950. The "7" refers to Lithium's atomic mass. Prescription lithium is available as lithium citrate syrup but is usually dispensed as lithium carbonate tablets or capsules.

FDA-approved in 1970, lithium is the only mood stabilizer that is not an antiepileptic. Antiepileptics raise seizure threshold. Lithium modestly decreases seizure threshold, making seizures slightly more likely to occur.

Lithium is neuroprotective, i.e., keeps neurons from dying. It is arguably an essential trace nutrient for mental wellbeing. Small amounts of lithium are present in vegetables and drinking water. Higher amounts of naturally occurring lithium in drinking water have been associated with decreased rates of suicide and violent crime (GN Schrauzer et al, 1990). Lithium has been shown to extend healthy lifespan of *Drosophila* fruit flies by about 8% (Castillo-Quan et al, 2016). Long-term exposure to low dose lithium appears to promote longevity in humans (Zarse et al, 2011). Lithium is an effective treatment for Alzheimer's disease (Mauer et al, 2014) and might prevent pre-dementia from progressing to Alzheimer's disease (Forlenza et al, 2011). The mechanism of neuroprotection and mood stabilization appears to involve brain-derived neurotrophic factor (BDNF).

Lithium is a first-line add-on for treatment-resistant unipolar depression, usually at a low to moderate dose. 68% of depressed patients over age 65 responded to lithium augmentation, improving faster than younger individuals. 47% of those < 65 responded (Buspavanich et al, 2019). Lithium is used off-label for prevention of migraine, cluster, and vascular headaches. Lithium increases white blood cell (WBC) count, making it a treatment option for neutropenia, including clozapine-induced neutropenia. Lithium inhibits antidiuretic hormone (ADH) and can be used to counter syndrome of inappropriate ADH secretion (SIADH).

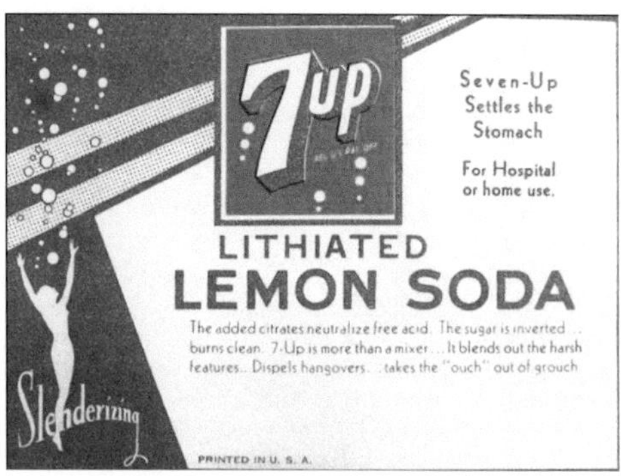

7-up contained lithium until 1950

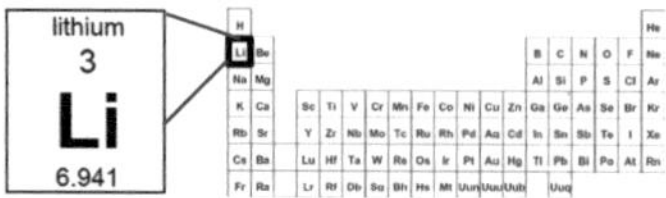

Lithium is renally cleared, unmetabolized. As an element, there is nothing it could be metabolized to. Therefore it is not involved in CYP enzyme interactions. Lithium is subject to kinetic interactions when other drugs affect the rate of lithium clearance by the kidneys. Lithium has a narrow therapeutic index, i.e., the toxic range is not far from the therapeutic range. A **black box warning** advises to start lithium only if a facility is available for prompt serum level testing. Signs of lithium toxicity include tremor, diarrhea, vomiting, abdominal pain, weakness, and sedation. Consequences of lithium toxicity may include renal damage, seizure, and coma.

Although toxic lithium levels can result in cardiac conduction delays, at therapeutic doses lithium is cardioprotective and lowers the risk of myocardial infarction. Lithium does not increase risk of stroke, which cannot be said of carbamazepine (Chen et al, 2019).

To avoid lithium toxicity, patients should be advised to avoid NSAIDS (ibuprofen, naproxen) and instead use aspirin or acetaminophen for pain. Patients should also remind their other doctors that they are on lithium, especially when diuretics or blood pressure medications are discussed. The most significant contributors to lithium toxicity are NSAIDS and thiazide diuretics, including hydrochlorothiazide (HCTZ) and chlorthalidone. See page 26 for the full list of "battery chargers" that increase lithium levels (ACE inhibitors, ARBs, metronidazole, etc).

Lithium side effects are dose-dependent, including weight gain, fine tremor, acne, excessive thirst, and frequent urination. If thirst and polyuria are extreme, the cause may be lithium-induced nephrogenic diabetes insipidus (deficient response by kidneys to ADH). If nausea is a problem, reduce dose or switch to Lithium ER (Lithobid). Otherwise, immediate-release lithium is preferable for maintenance treatment. Taking the entire daily dose of immediate-release lithium at bedtime reduces polyuria and decreases the risk of renal problems (Gitlin et al, 2016) by giving the kidneys a break during daytime.

Lithium increases the incidence of hypothyroidism 6-fold. Since about 15% of lithium-treated patients will become hypothyroid, TSH should be monitored routinely so levothyroxine (Synthroid) can be added if TSH gets high. Renal function needs to be monitored with a metabolic panel (BMP or CMP). When lithium is combined with a 1st generation antipsychotic, extrapyramidal symptoms (EPS) and neuroleptic malignant syndrome (NMS) may be more likely, which is considered a neurotoxic effect of unknown mechanism. Rarely, lithium may contribute to serotonin syndrome. For individuals over age 50, it is recommended to get an EKG prior to starting (standard dose) lithium because arrhythmias are possible. Very rarely lithium is associated with intracranial hypertension (pseudotumor cerebri), which presents as headache and ringing in the ears with heartbeats. If untreated, intracranial hypertension can lead to loss of vision.

When taken during the first trimester of pregnancy, lithium poses a low risk (1 in 1,500) of Ebstein's anomaly, a cardiac condition involving the tricuspid valve. Lithium is certainly less teratogenic than valproic acid (Depakote, Depakene) or carbamazepine (Tegretol). Lithium is considered safe for fetal development after the first trimester, but maintaining steady lithium levels during pregnancy and after delivery is challenging. Lithium concentration of fetal blood is equal to that of maternal blood with levels continually decreasing in the first and second trimesters, risking subtherapeutic concentration. Lithium concentration gradually increases in the third trimester and in the postpartum, risking toxicity. If lithium is continued during pregnancy, levels should be checked weekly.

In 2019 the FDA lowered the approved minimum age for lithium from 12 to 7 years.

Lithium works well in combination with valproic acid (Depakote, Depakene), lamotrigine (Lamictal), and second generation antipsychotics (SGAs).

With lithium treatment (at standard doses), it is necessary to monitor blood levels. As for any drug, blood levels should be checked at "trough", which is about 12 hours after the last dose. For treatment of acute mania, a relatively high level of 1.0 to 1.4 mmol/L is desired. Once mood has stabilized, the maintenance dose should be decreased to achieve a level of 0.6 to 1.0 mmol/L.. For augmentation of treatment-resistant depression (TRD), the recommended target serum level is 0.5–0.8 mmol/L. A level of 2.0 mmol/L is considered toxic. Discontinuation of lithium is ideally accomplished by slow taper over about 6–12 weeks.

It could be argued that there is no such thing as a subtherapeutic lithium level. Some naturopathic doctors recommend tiny dose 5–20 mg (equivalent) lithium orotate capsules as a nutritional supplement. These capsules are available over-the-counter (OTC) at health food stores and on Amazon.com.

Tremor is a telltale sign that lithium level may be too high. If tremor occurs at therapeutic blood level, consider adding low dose propranolol (about 20 mg TID), which is effective treatment for many types of tremor.

Heavy sweating (for a healthy and adequately hydrated individual) may decrease lithium levels, because sweat-to-serum ratio for lithium exceeds that for sodium by a factor of 4 (Jefferson et al, 1982). Dehydration, however, can contribute to lithium toxicity and renal insufficiency.

Five strengths of lithium

Strength	Purpose	Blood level (mmol/L)	Approximate total daily dose	Status	Comments
	Acute mania	1.0–1.4	1,200–1,800 mg	FDA-approved	For acute mania, start at least 300 mg TID of extended-release Lithium ER (Lithobid). Adjust dose every 3 days based on response and blood level. Consider using the ER formulation initially to minimize side effects. Transition to a lower dose of immediate-release lithium (caps or tabs) preferably dosed entirely at night, which is easier on the kidneys.
	Maintenance of bipolar disorder	0.6–1.0	900–1,200 mg	FDA-approved	For an outpatient who is not acutely manic, one strategy is to start Lithium ER or IR 300 mg HS x 5 days, then 600 mg HS x 5 days, then 900 mg HS. Adjust dose based on blood level, and transition to immediate-release lithium (Eskalith) dosed entirely at night.
	Treatment resistant depression	0.5–0.8	600 mg	Off-label	Lithium is one of the most effective adjuncts to an antidepressant for refractory depression. Consider starting Lithium ER (Lithobid) 300 mg BID and transitioning to 600 mg Lithium IR (Eskalith) at bedtime.
	Neuroprotection; Dementia; Suicide prevention; Headaches	0.1–0.4	150–300 mg	Off-label	The author is a big fan of low-dose lithium 150–300 mg HS for anyone at risk of committing suicide. The rationale is that lithium has been proven to prevent suicide and prevent dementia, so why not prescribe a neuroprotective dose that is safe and has no expected side effects? Monitoring of lithium level is entirely unnecessary at the 150 mg dose, and probably unnecessary at the 300 mg dose unless the patient has side effects or is taking a battery charger (see next page). TSH and renal function should be monitored for all patients.
	Nutritional supplement	< 0.1	5–60 mg	Off-label/ Over-the-counter	Since trace lithium in drinking water has been shown to prevent suicide, some naturopaths recommend tiny dose over-the-counter lithium as an "essential trace nutrient" for mental wellbeing. See below for dosing options.

Microdose lithium pills are available on Amazon as 5, 10, and 20 mg (equivalent) capsules of lithium orotate, costing about $4–$10 monthly. 130 mg of lithium orotate is equivalent to 5 mg of elemental lithium. Lithium orotate is not available by prescription. 60 mg of daily lithium can be accomplished with prescription lithium citrate liquid, which is 300 mg (equivalent) per 5 mL. So, 1 mg of liquid would be 60 mg daily. If you prescribe a 500 mL bottle, it will last for over a year. Less precise tiny doses could be accomplished by chopping 300 mg lithium carbonate tablets into tiny pieces.

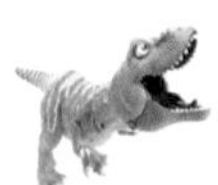

Dynamic interactions:

- CNS depression
- Decreased seizure threshold
- Serotonergic (mild)
- Decreased ability of antidiuretic hormone (ADH), vasopressin (AVP), and desmopressin (DDAVP) to concentrate urine
- Nephrotoxicity

Idiosyncratic interactions (unknown mechanism, rare):

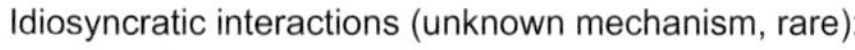

- Increased risk of extrapyramidal effects (EPS) with first generation antipsychotics (FGAs)
- Neurotoxicity when combined with verapamil (calcium channel blocker)
- Neurotoxicity when combined with carbamazepine (Tegretol)

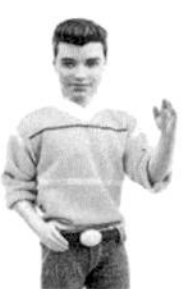

Kinetic interactions (illustrated on the next page)

- Enhanced renal excretion of lithium in alkaline urine, as caused by carbonic anhydrase inhibitors such as acetazolamide (Diamox), topiramate (Topamax), and zonisamide (Zonegran)
- Enhanced renal excretion of lithium by osmotic diuretics such as mannitol
- Enhanced renal excretion of lithium by methylxanthines such as caffeine and theophylline, which are mild diuretics
- Decreased renal excretion by the "battery chargers" (shown on the next page) may result in lithium toxicity; most often with NSAIDS and thiazide diuretics
- Interferes with production of thyroid hormone

Lithium kinetic interactions
involving renal clearance

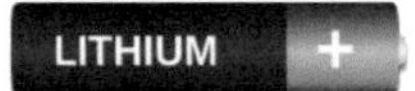

Lithium is removed from the body almost exclusively by the kidneys. Several medications affect the rate of lithium clearance. Since lithium has a narrow therapeutic index, blood levels need to be closely followed.

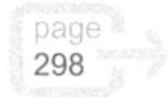

Serum lithium levels are mildly **decreased** by:

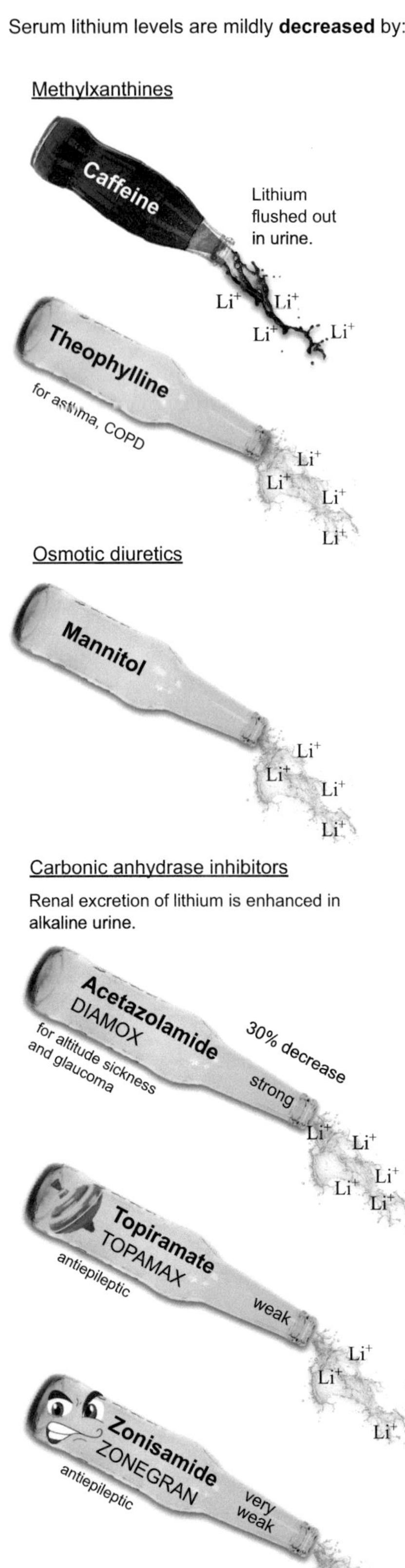

Lithium levels are **increased** by:

Thiazide Diuretics

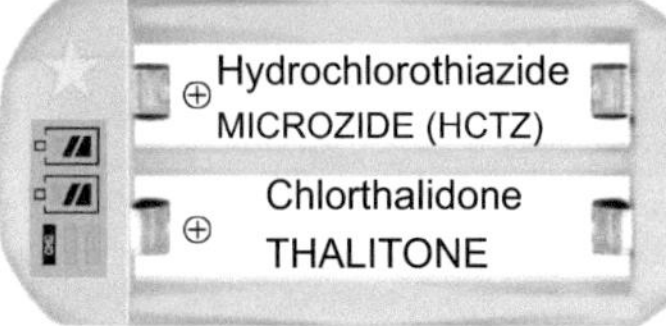

Increased lithium reabsorption

ACE Inhibitors "-prils"

Angiotensin-converting enzyme inhibitors

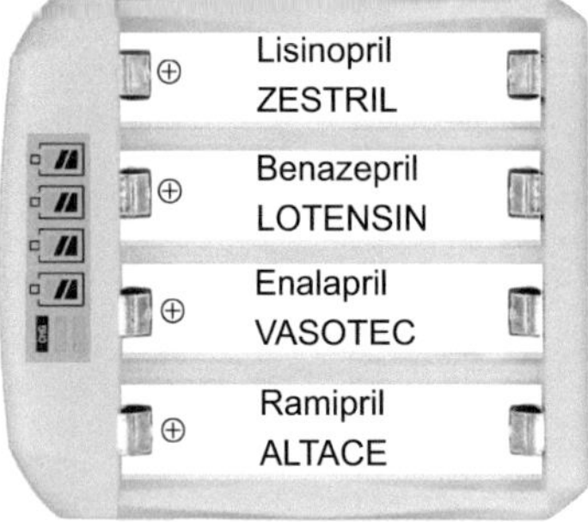

ARBs "-sartans"

Angiotensin II receptor blockers

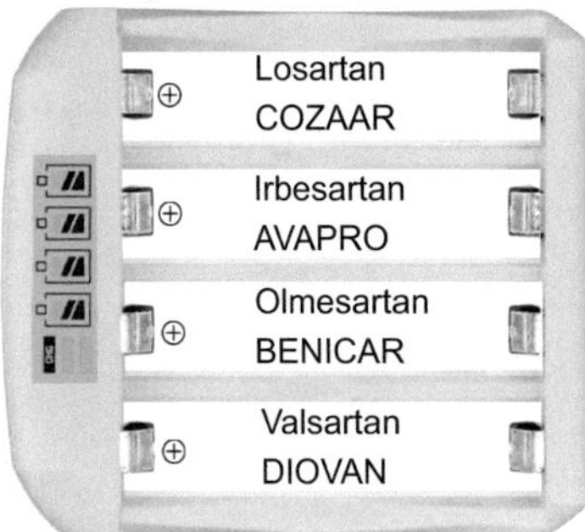

NSAIDs

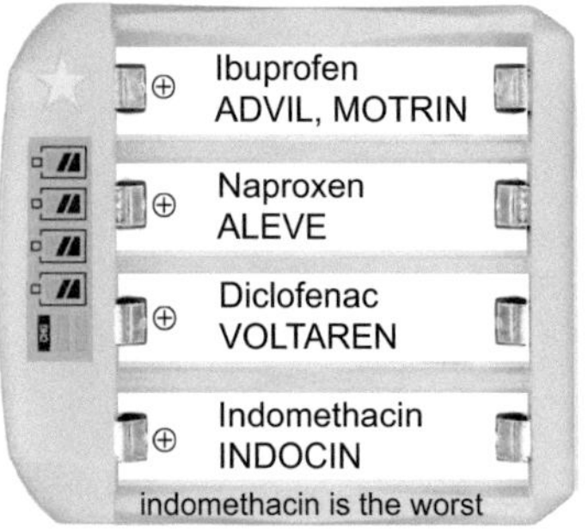

Also:
etodolac
fenoprofen
ketoprofen
ketorolac
nabumetone
oxaprozin
piroxicam
meclofenamate

Not:
sulindac
aspirin

COX-2 inhibitor

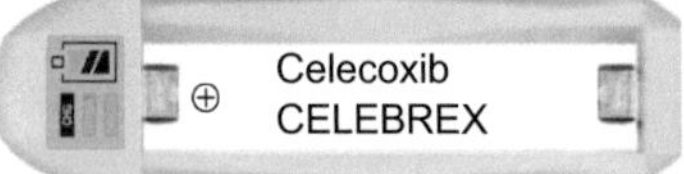

☆ Thiazide diuretics and NSAIDS have the greatest potential to increase lithium concentrations, usually 25% to 40%. Rarely the increase may be much greater, leading to lithium toxicity. If another prescriber insists on adding a thiazide or NSAID, a reasonable approach is to decrease lithium dose by about 30% and recheck blood level in one week.

Tetracyclines

Antibiotics

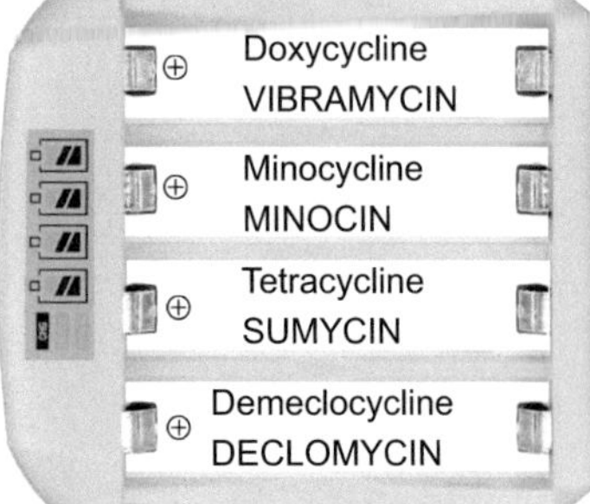

Antimicrobial

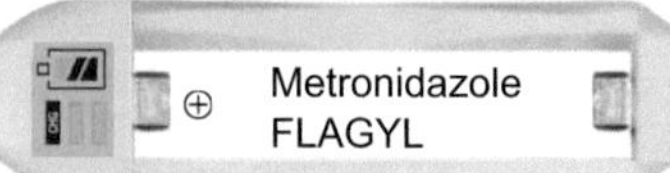

Lithium levels are **not** significantly affected by:

Loop diuretics
- Furosemide (LASIX)
- Bumetanide (BUMEX)

Potassium-sparing diuretics
- Spironolactone (ALDACTONE)
- Amiloride (MIDAMOR)
- Triamterene (DYRENIUM)

Calcium channel blockers
- Amlodipine (NORVASC)
- Diltiazem (CARDIZEM)
- Verapamil (CALAN)
- Nifedipine (PROCARDIA)

Central alpha agonists
- Clonidine (CATAPRES)
- Guanfacine (TENEX)

Beta blockers
- Metoprolol (LOPRESSOR)
- Atenolol (TENORMIN)
- Propranolol (INDERAL)
- Labetalol (TRANDATE)
- Nebivolol (BYSTOLIC)
- Bisoprolol (ZEBETA)
- Nadolol (CORGARD)

Vasodilators
- Hydralazine (APRESOLINE)
- Isosorbide mononitrate (IMDUR)

Pain medications
- Aspirin (BAYER, EXCEDRIN)
- Sulindac (NSAID)
- Acetaminophen (TYLENOL)
- Tramadol (ULTRAM)
- Opioids

Conclusion: Educate patients that NSAIDS, blood pressure meds, and diuretics can cause lithium toxicity. For OTC pain medications, they should choose Tylenol or aspirin. Advise them to inform the prescriber if they are planning to change their caffeine intake. Excedrin is OK (combo of aspirin, acetaminophen, and caffeine). Check lithium levels frequently for patients on interacting medications. Teach the signs of lithium toxicity including tremor, nausea, diarrhea, fatigue, and drowsiness.

New AEDs are often initially approved as adjuncts for focal seizures (formerly called partial seizures) but are prescribed off-label for adjunctive treatment of bilateral tonic-clonic seizures (formerly primary generalized seizures) and/or as monotherapy. GABA is the brain's principal inhibitory neurotransmitter. AEDs with "gab" in their name are either structurally related to GABA and/or lead to GABA(A) receptor activation. Several benzodiazepines (Chapter 4) are approved for epilepsy but are excluded from this list. Phenobarbital and primidone are barbiturates, featured in Chapter 3.

The monographs in this chapter are presented in order of mood stabilizers followed by the non-mood stabilizing AEDs in descending order of popularity in terms of number of prescriptions issued (Rx #).

Rx #	AED	~ Cost	Psychiatric uses	Comments
#1	Gabapentin (NEURONTIN)	$10	Pain, Anxiety, Alcoholism	#13 prescribed drug overall, usually for indications other than seizure disorder including neuropathic pain, fibromyalgia, and restless legs syndrome (RLS)
#2	Lamotrigine (LAMICTAL)	$10	1st line mood stabilizer	#70 overall. First-line for bipolar maintenance and seizure disorders because of relative safety and benign side effect profile; Dose must be titrated over 5 weeks to avoid Stevens-Johnson Syndrome (SJS). Broad spectrum AED
#3	Pregabalin (LYRICA)	$100	Anxiety	#83 overall; FDA-approved for focal seizures (adjunct), neuropathic pain, fibromyalgia, and post-herpetic neuralgia; Schedule V controlled substance (least restrictive); Similar to gabapentin; Approved for generalized anxiety in the UK
#4	Topiramate (TOPAMAX)	$10	Bipolar adjunct, weight loss, alcoholism, PTSD	#85 overall; Commonly causes (reversible) cognitive impairment at doses ≥ 200 mg; 15% risk of renal stones and possible metabolic acidosis, both attributable to alkalinization of urine
#5	Levetiracetam (KEPPRA)	$15	No!	#89 overall; Broad spectrum AED, often first-line for epilepsy; High incidence of irritability and mood disturbance, with potential for suicidal ideation, psychosis, and aggression
#6	Divalproex DR (DEPAKOTE)	$15	1st line mood stabilizer	#129 overall; The active drug is valproic acid (VPA). Potential for hepatotoxicity, hyperammonemic encephalopathy, tremor, and polycystic ovary syndrome (PCOS)
#7	Carbamazepine (TEGRETOL)	$40	2nd line mood stabilizer	#197 overall; Shredder CYP inDucer (Page 7); Several serious health risks; Narrow spectrum AED
#8	Phenytoin (DILANTIN)	$25	No	#201 overall; Shredder CYP inDucer that decreases blood levels of countless co-administered drugs; May cause gingival hypertrophy, coarse facial features, nystagmus, and cognitive impairment; Blood level monitoring is required; Narrow spectrum AED
#9	Primidone (MYSOLINE)	$15	No	#237 overall; This barbiturate is metabolized to phenobarbital. Off-label treatment of tremor; Not a controlled substance
#10	Oxcarbazepine (TRILEPTAL)	$20	2nd line mood stabilizer	#244 overall; Similar to carbamazepine with fewer risks and fewer interactions, but with greater risk of hyponatremia
#11	Phenobarbital (LUMINAL)	$30	Alcohol detox	Schedule IV controlled barbiturate; The oldest AED still in use, discovered in 1912; For anxiety treatment, barbiturates have been replaced by the safer benzodiazepines
#12	Zonisamide (ZONEGRAN)	$20	Alcoholism, Nightmares	May cause irritability and cognitive impairment; Rare incidence of psychosis; May cause weight loss; Broad spectrum AED
#13	Lacosamide (VIMPAT)	$900	No	Schedule V controlled substance (least restrictive) due to possible euphoria; Low incidence of mood problems; Narrow spectrum AED; Off patent in 2022
#14	Ethosuximide (ZARONTIN)	$100	No	Used only for petit mal (absence) seizures; Rarely associated with psychotic behavior; Risk of Stevens-Johnson syndrome (SJS)
#15	Eslicarbazepine (APTIOM)	$1000	No (due to cost)	Prodrug of an active metabolite of oxcarbazepine; Risk of hyponatremia and Stevens-Johnson syndrome; Off patent in 2021; Potential mood stabilizer
#16	Rufinamide (BANZEL)	$1000	Experimental for bipolar	Approved in 2008 as an adjunct for Lennox-Gastaut syndrome, but has potential as a broad spectrum AED; Can shorten QT interval
#17	Felbamate (FELBATOL)	$200	No	Considered relatively benign in terms of psychiatric adverse effects. Broad spectrum AED; Small risk of aplastic anemia and hepatic failure
#18	Brivaracetam (BRIVIACT)	$1000	No!	Analog of levetiracetam; Less likely to cause disturbance of mood/behavior than levetiracetam; Schedule V controlled (least restrictive)
#19	Tiagabine (GABITRIL)	$100	Mood stabilization and anxiety	GABA reuptake inhibitor; increases percentage of slow wave sleep; Can interfere with color perception; May *induce* seizures in patients without epilepsy
#20	Perampanel (FYCOMPA)	$500	No!	AMPA receptor antagonist; Schedule III controlled; **Black box warnings** for severe psychiatric and behavioral reactions including hostility, aggression, and homicidal ideation—*"Fight-compa"*
#21	Vigabatrin (SABRIL)	$4000	No!	Blocks breakdown of GABA; Restricted distribution due to risk of vision loss; May cause irritability, depression, and confusion; Narrow spectrum AED
NEW 2020	Cenobamate (XCOPRI)	$1000	No	Slow titration over 11 weeks is necessary to avoid Drug Reaction with Eosinophilia and Systemic Symptoms (DRESS).

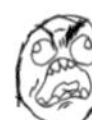

An angry face means that a medication may cause significant irritability and potentially aggression, to the extent it should not be used as a mood stabilizer. Be aware almost any psychotropic drug has a potential for irritability with certain individuals.

#70
1994
$3–$67

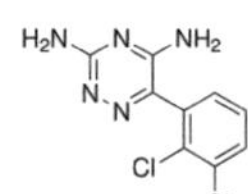

Lamotrigine (LAMICTAL)

lah MO tre jeen / lah MIK tal

"Lamb ictal"

- Antiepileptic
- Voltage-gated sodium and calcium channel blocker
- Glutamate ⇩

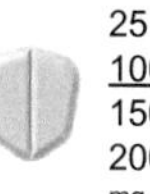

25
100
150
200
mg

FDA-approved for:
- Bipolar I maintenance
- Focal seizures
- Lennox-Gastaut syndrome
- Bilateral tonic-clonic seizures

Used off-label for:
- Bipolar II maintenance
- Major depressive disorder
- Borderline personality disorder
- Neuropathic pain
- Fibromyalgia
- PTSD
- Other seizure disorders

Lamotrigine is the mood stabilizer of choice for maintenance of bipolar disorder. Lamotrigine has few health risks and few side effects. The most commonly reported side effects at high doses are dizziness and blurred vision. Lamotrigine does not cause weight gain and is generally non-sedating. No lab monitoring is required. It is the most effective stabilizer for preventing bipolar depressive episodes and has been demonstrated to be effective for unipolar depression.

Lamictal is of no use for an acute manic episode because the dose must be slowly titrated over 5 weeks to avoid life-threatening skin reactions including Stevens-Johnson syndrome (SJS) and toxic epidermal necrolysis (TEN). Lamotrigine should be stopped immediately in the event of a serious dermatologic reaction. Notwithstanding the risk of SJS, lamotrigine is one of the safest psychotropic medications. It is nontoxic in overdose. Dose is determined by clinical response rather than serum levels. If a lamotrigine level is ordered, results may take a week because local laboratories must send the blood sample to an outside lab.

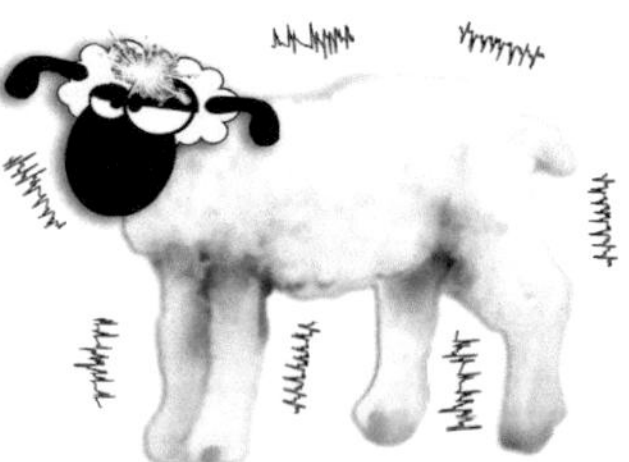

"Ictal" refers to a neurologic event such as a seizure.

Lamotrigine has some unique aspects. Among several mechanisms of actions, it blocks the release of glutamate, the brain's principal excitatory neurotransmitter. Lamotrigine is a broad-spectrum AED, effective for several types of seizures.

Stevens-Johnson syndrome (SJS)	Benign rash
❖ Usually occurs between 1–12 weeks ❖ Purpuric (non-blanching), may be tender ❖ Rapidly confluent and wide-spread ❖ Usually involves neck and above ❖ Can involve conjunctiva, mucous membranes ❖ With fever, malaise or lymphadenopathy ❖ Leukocytosis	❖ Peaks at 10–14 days ❖ Non-tender ❖ Spotty (non-confluent) ❖ Below the neck ❖ No involvement of mucous membranes ❖ No fever, malaise or lymphadenopathy ❖ Normal CBC and CMP

High dose lamotrigine can shorten QT interval, which does not pose a clinical risk, except in the case of familial short QT syndrome or in combination with other QT-shortening drugs such as rufinamide (Banzel), digoxin or magnesium. Contrast this with the many psychotropic medications that prolong QT interval.

Before lamotrigine became generically available, three Lamictal starter packs were available to address these interactions:

Starter pack	For those taking	Pack contains	Standard titration	Max Dose
Orange pack	No interacting medications	5 week supply = 25 mg tabs #42, 100 mg tabs #7	25 mg QD x 2 wks, then 50 mg x 2 wk, then 100 mg x 1 wk. The usual maintenance dose starting on week six is **200 mg** dosed AM, HS or divided 100 mg BID.	400 mg total (200 mg BID)
Blue (half strength)	Valproate (Depakote) Valproic acid (Depakene)	5 wk supply = 25 mg tabs #35	25 mg every other day x 2 wk, then 25 mg QD x 2 wk, then 50 mg QD x 1 wk. Usual maintenance dose starting week six is **100 mg QD**.	200 mg total (100 mg BID)
Green (double strength)	Carbamazepine (Tegretol), Phenytoin (Dilantin), Phenobarbital (Luminal) or Primidone (Mysoline)	5 wk supply = 25 mg tabs #84 100 mg tabs #14	50 mg QD x 2 wk, then 50 mg BID x 2 wk, then 100 mg BID x 1 wk,then 150 mg BID x 1 wk. Usual maintenance dose is **200 mg BID** starting week 6.	700 mg total (350 mg BID)

Lamotrigine is principally metabolized by UDP-glucuronosyltransferase (UGT) in the liver, as in "U Got Tagged!" (conjugated) with glucuronic acid. Specifically, UGT1A4 is the most relevant UGT enzyme. CYP450 enzymes are not involved. Lamotrigine is not an inducer or inhibitor of other drugs, and is only a victim (vulnerable substrate) in a small number of kinetic interactions.

Dynamic interactions:
- Sedation/CNS depression (uncommon)
- Shortening of QT interval (at high dose)

Kinetic interactions:
- UGT substrate

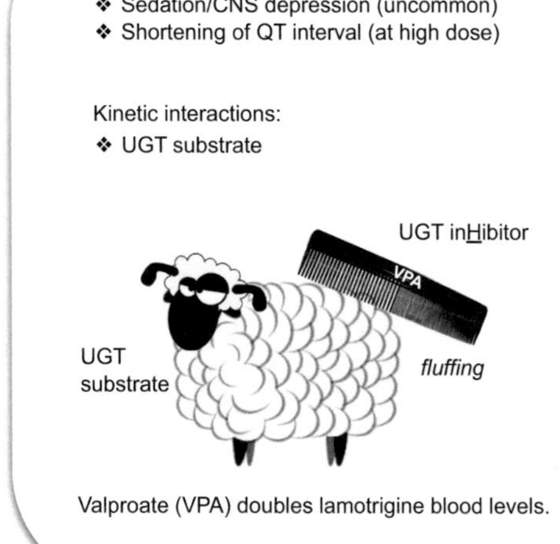

Valproate (VPA) doubles lamotrigine blood levels.

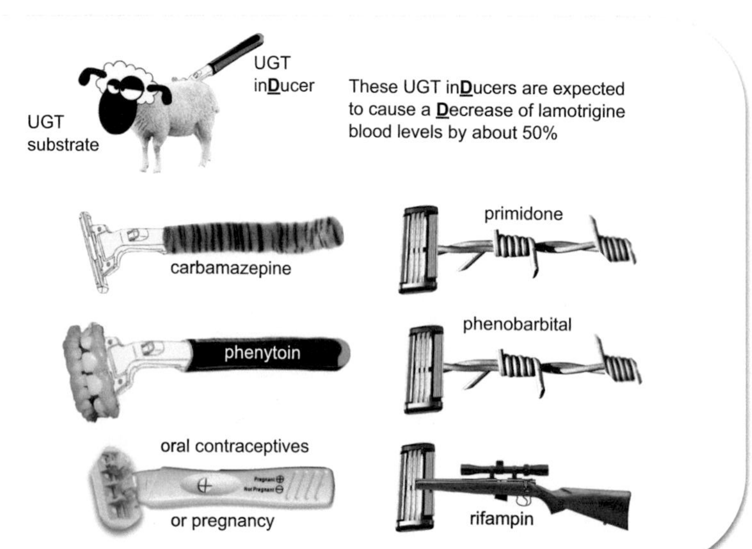

These UGT inDucers are expected to cause a Decrease of lamotrigine blood levels by about 50%

1962
$26–$83 caps
$21–$68 liquid

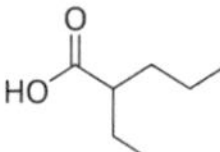

Valproic Acid (DEPAKENE)

val PROE ik / DEP a keen

"Dip a Keno (ball in) acid"

- ❖ Antiepileptic
- ❖ Voltage-gated sodium channel blocker
- ❖ Glutamate ⇩

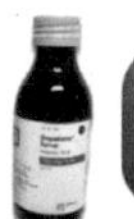

250 mg liquid-filled caps

FDA-approved for:

- ❖ Bipolar disorder, acute mania
- ❖ Focal impaired awareness seizure
- ❖ Absence seizures
- ❖ Migraine prophylaxis

Used off-label for:

- ❖ Bipolar maintenance
- ❖ Aggression (drug of choice)
- ❖ Lennox-Gastaut syndrome (1st line)

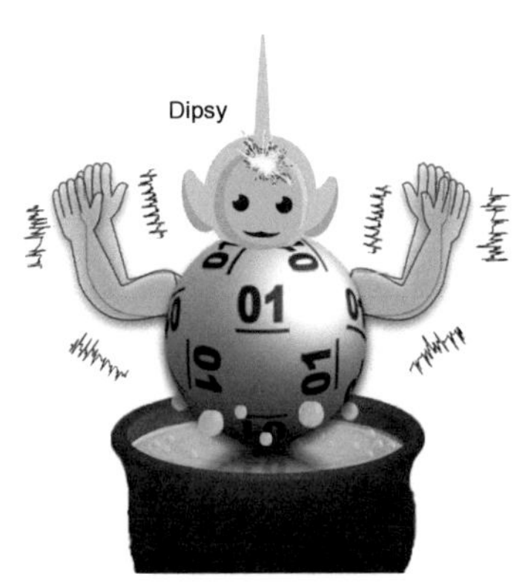

Forms of valproate:

page 30

Valproic acid (VPA) DEPAKENE	Divalproex DEPAKOTE
The active drug, of which serum levels are monitored	The most commonly prescribed form of valproate (see next page)

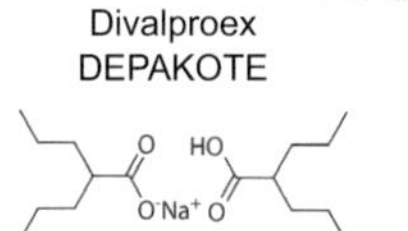

Valproate (available as valproic acid and divalproex) is the drug of choice for acute mania. Depakene is the pure form of VPA, available as liquid filled capsules and oral solution. Depakene caps are uncommonly prescribed, because Depakene causes more gastrointestinal upset than divalproex (Depakote). Depakene oral solution is used for patients prone to cheeking pills to collect or surreptitiously dispose of them. The most common complaint patients have about VPA is feeling sedated.

Depakene may be more effective than Depakote for mania. Wassef et al (2005) found that hospital stays were 32.7% longer for those started on Depakote (over Depakene). For those patients started on Depakene, only 6.4% had to be switched to Depakote due to GI distress.

VPA has several **black box warnings** including hepatotoxicity, pancreatitis (including fatal hemorrhagic pancreatitis), and teratogenicity (neural tube defects, autism, low IQ). The teratogenicity of VPA is partially due to depletion of folate. VPA is also less than ideal for women of childbearing age due to fetal risks and 10% risk of polycystic ovary syndrome (PCOS).

VPA may elevate ammonia levels, which may lead to hyperammonemic encephalopathy. Ammonia level should be checked if there are mental status changes. Since hyperammonemia is dose-related, it may resolve when Depakote dose is reduced. Hepatotoxicity is a rare idiosyncratic reaction that is not dose-related, with most cases occurring within 3 months. With VPA, asymptomatic increase of liver enzymes is not necessarily indicative of hepatic dysfunction. It is also possible to have hyperammonemia without elevated liver enzymes.

VPA is approved for acute manic episodes, not for bipolar maintenance. Although it is effective for preventing relapse of mood episodes and is effective for rapid cycling, VPA is less than ideal for bipolar maintenance due to side effects. 50% of patients gain > 10% body weight. Tremor can be severe for some patients. Over 20% develop reversible thrombocytopenia at high-end doses. VPA may rarely cause edema.

VPA can cause hair loss, which can be remedied with supplementation of zinc 30 mg, selenium 200 mcg, and biotin 10 mg daily, taken at a different time than VPA (which interferes with their absorption). Chelated zinc is easier on the stomach. Hair loss stops when VPA is stopped.

VPA is metabolized in the liver with CYP450 enzymes only playing a minimal role, so it has relatively few drug-drug interactions. The lack of kinetic interactions is a major advantage of VPA over the "shredder" carbamazepine (Tegretol). VPA doubles lamotrigine (Lamictal) levels by inHibiting UGT (phase II metabolism). There is increased risk of encephalopathy if VPA is coadministered with topiramate (Topamax).

VPA is highly protein bound. Only unbound (free) VPA is active. When coadministered with high dose aspirin (which is also highly protein bound), the percentage of free VPA will increase and Depakene will be stronger than suggested by the standard VPA level (total VPA). If the patient has low albumin, the percentage of free VPA will be predictably higher.

Dosing: Initial dosing is the same as Depakote (see next page). Maintenance dose is guided by VPA blood levels. The active medication that is monitored through the standard blood test is total valproic acid (VPA). The therapeutic range for bipolar disorder is officially defined as 50 to 125 μg/mL. For acute mania, aim for VPA level of 80–120 μg/mL. For bipolar maintenance, shoot for 50–100 μg/mL. Over 150 μg/mL is considered toxic. For migraine prophylaxis start 500 mg x 1 week, then 1,000 mg. See above for situations where ordering a free VPA level may be indicated. If used long-term, add folic acid (folate) 0.4 mg daily, which is depleted by VPA.

Dynamic interactions:

- ❖ Sedative/CNS depression
- ❖ Hyponatremia
- ❖ Hyperammonemia
- ❖ Antiplatelet effects

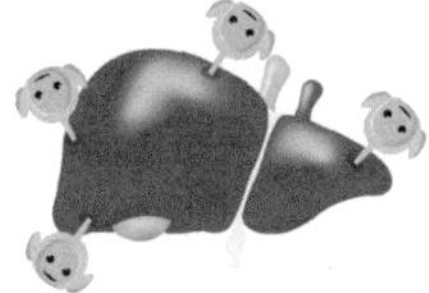

VPA can cause hepatotoxicity

Kinetic interactions:

- ❖ VPA is highly protein bound. Only the unbound fraction is active. High dose aspirin or low serum albumin will make Depakene stronger than suggested by serum total VPA level, because a high percentage of VPA is unbound (active).
- ❖ 2C9 substrate (minor)
- ❖ UGT1A4 inHibitor – can double lamotrigine (Lamictal) blood levels
- ❖ UGT2B15 inHibitor – can double blood levels of "LOT" benzos (lorazepam, oxazepam, temazepam)

page 13

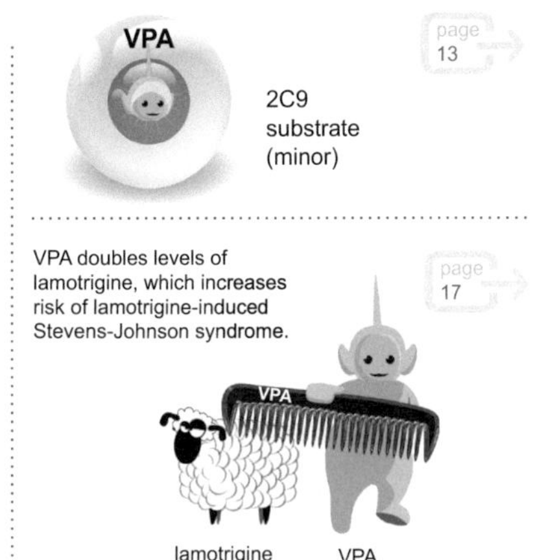

page 17

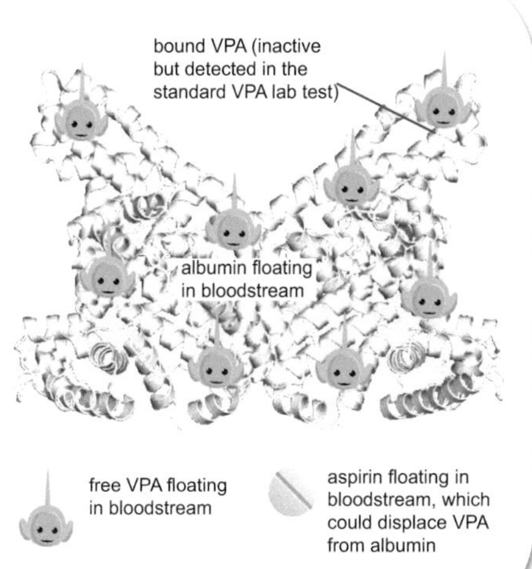

#129
1996
$14–$128

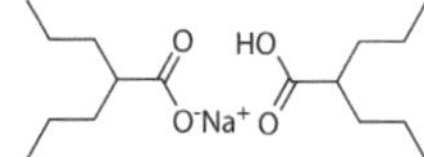

Divalproex (DEPAKOTE)

dye val PRO ex / DEP a kote

"Dip-a-Coat"

❖ Antiepileptic
❖ Voltage-gated sodium channel blocker
❖ Glutamate ⇩

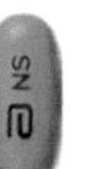

125
250
500
mg

Indications:

❖ See Depakene monograph on preceding page.

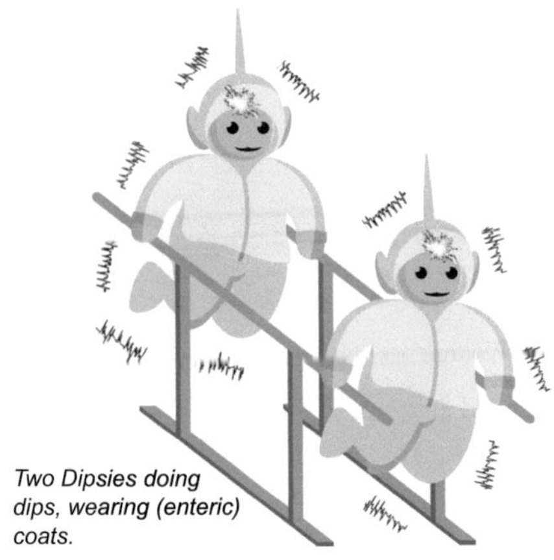

Two Dipsies doing dips, wearing (enteric) coats.

Divalproex is a compound formed by adding sodium hydroxide to two valproic acid (VPA) molecules, yielding a molecule that is double the size of Depakene. In the small intestine divalproex is broken down to the two molecules of VPA.

Depakote is the enteric "koted" form of VPA that causes less gastrointestinal upset. Depakote and Depakene are bioequivalent per mg dose. The VPA of Depakote is absorbed more slowly than Depakene. Because of this, Depakote is described as a "delayed-release" (DR) version of VPA.

"Regular" Depakote is listed in ePrescribe systems as Depakote DR (delayed-release), intended for BID dosing. There is no "Depakote IR" (immediate-release) because that would be Depakene (straight valproic acid). When the doctor orders Depakote, "Depakote DR is what the doctor ordered".

Dosing: A reasonable starting dose for bipolar mania is a minimum of 10 mg/pound split BID. Although Depakote DR it is intended for BID dosing, some doctors prescribe the entire daily dose of Depakote DR at bedtime to enhance compliance and minimize side effects. For migraine prophylaxis start 500 mg x 1 week, then 1,000 mg. If used long-term, add folic acid (folate) 0.4 mg daily, which is depleted by VPA. Refer to the Depakene monograph on the preceding page for the basic information about this drug, target blood levels, and situations where ordering a free VPA level may be indicated.

Dynamic interactions:

❖ Sedative/CNS depression
❖ Hyponatremia
❖ Hyperammonemia
❖ Antiplatelet effects

Kinetic interactions:

❖ VPA is highly protein bound. Only the unbound fraction is active. High dose aspirin or low serum albumin will make Depakote stronger than suggested by serum total VPA level, because a high percentage of VPA is unbound (active).
❖ 2C9 substrate (minor)
❖ UGT inHibitor (refer to Depakene monograph on page 29) – can double blood levels of "LOT" benzos and lamotrigine

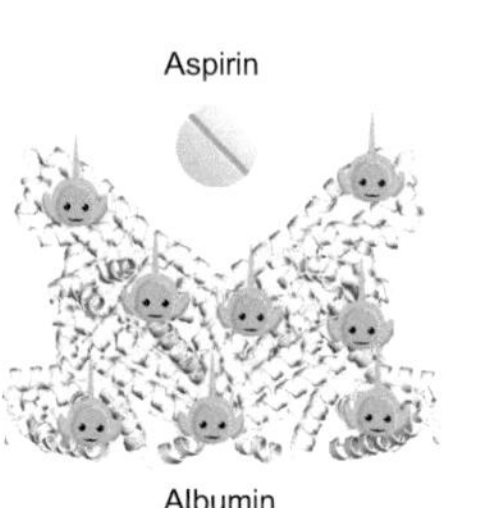

page 13

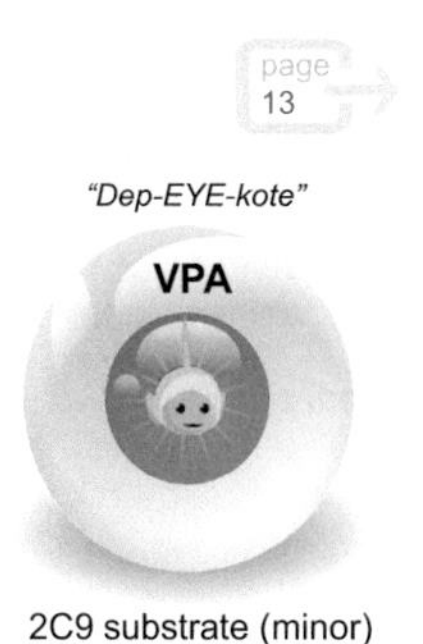

2C9 substrate (minor)

VPA doubles levels of lamotrigine

page 17

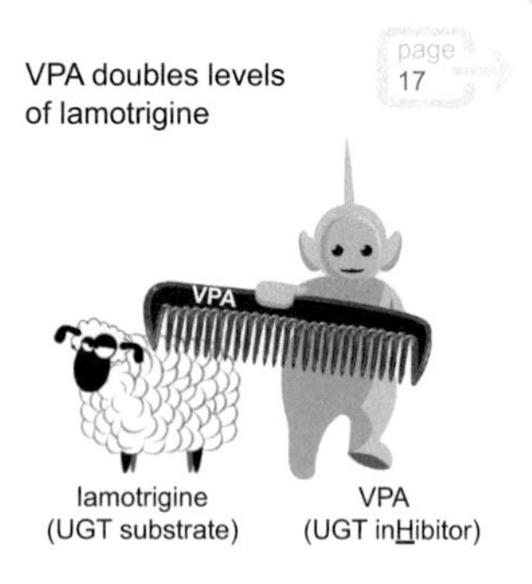

2000
$28–$229

Divalproex (DEPAKOTE ER)

di val pro ex / DEP a kote

"Dip-a-coat ER"

❖ Antiepileptic
❖ Voltage-gated sodium channel blocker
❖ Glutamate ⇩

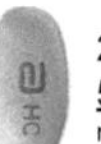

250
500
mg

Indications:

❖ See Depakene monograph on preceding page.

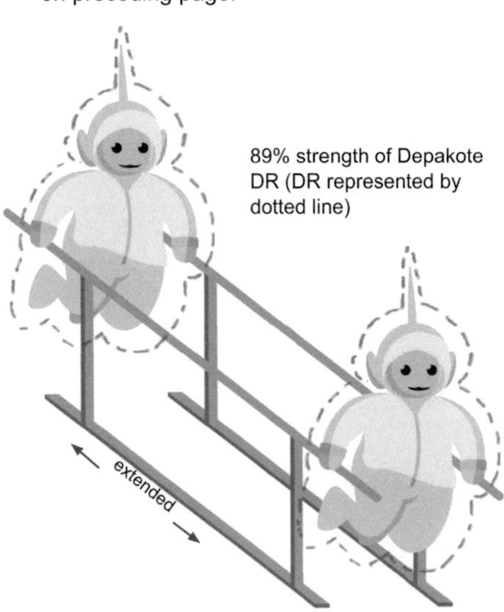

The once-daily formulation of divalproex is Depakote ER (extended-release). The label instructs to give it with food.

Regular Depakote (Depakote DR) and Depakote ER are not bioequivalent. Depakote ER delivers only about 89% of the VPA available by other formulations. It is baffling that Depakote DR is available in 125, 250, and 500 mg tabs and Depakote ER also comes in 250 and 500 mg tabs.

The ER formulation, intended for once daily dosing, costs twice as much as regular Depakote (DR). Many doctors prescribe regular Depakote (DR) once daily at bedtime anyhow. Think "Depakote ErroR"—the doctor may have ordered Depakote ER in error. If so, giving the ER formulation will lead to underdosing because Depakote ER has 89% bioavailability of the more commonly prescribed Depakote DR.

Depakote ER may have utility in certain situations, for instance when tapering off Depakote. There may be circumstances when it makes sense to change from DR to ER at the same dose to effect a slight reduction in strength.

Dosing: 89% bioequivalent to Depakote DR. The label instructs to "increase total daily dose by 8–20% if switching from DR to ER". For bipolar disorder, dose as you would with Depakote DR, but give the entire daily dose with the evening meal. The therapeutic range for bipolar disorder is officially defined as 50 to 125 µg/mL. For acute mania, aim for VPA level of 80–120 µg/mL. For bipolar maintenance, shoot for 50–100 µg/mL. Over 150 µg/mL is considered toxic. For migraine prophylaxis start 500 mg QD with food x 1 week, then 1,000 mg.

#197
1962
$23–$65

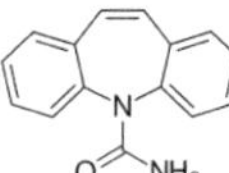

Carbamazepine (TEGRETOL)

kahr buh MAZ uh peen / TEG ra tal

"Tiger tail (in the) Car Maze"

- Antiepileptic
- Voltage-gated sodium channel blocker
- Glutamate ⇩

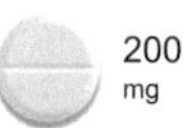

200 mg

FDA-approved for:
- Seizure disorder
- Trigeminal neuralgia
- Acute manic/mixed episode of bipolar I disorder (ER formulation)

Used off-label for:
- Bipolar maintenance
- Neuropathic pain
- Restless legs syndrome
- Migraine prophylaxis

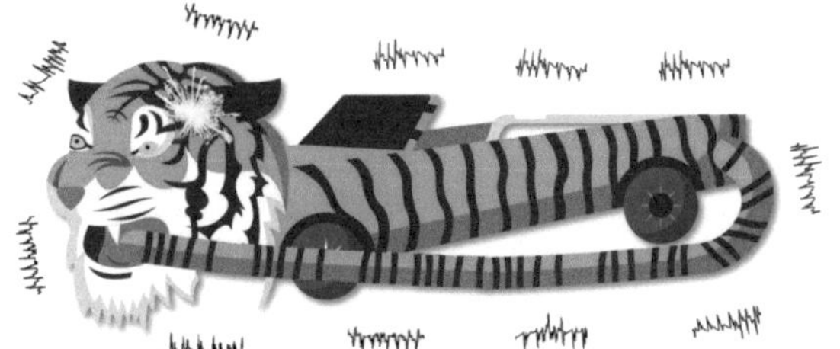

eating its own tail = in**D**ucing its own metabolism by CYP3A4 (auto-in**D**uction)

Risks of CBZ:

Terato-genicity

aplastic anemia (rare)

decreased bone mineral density

agranulo-cytosis (rare)

hyponatremia

Na⊕ Na⊕

hepatotoxicity

reduced levels of many medications

Carbamazepine (CBZ), released in 1962, is effective for bipolar mania but is considered second-line behind lithium and valproate. CBZ's usefulness is limited by drug-drug interactions. CBZ is a "shredder" in**D**ucer of multiple CYP enzymes, resulting in significantly **D**ecreased blood levels of a long list of medications. Always run an interaction check if CBZ is in the mix.

Carbamazepine even in**D**uces its own metabolism (CYP3A4). The effect occurs within 2 to 3 weeks (**D**elayed), then stabilizes. CBZ has an elimination half-life of 24 hours initially, then 15 hours after auto-induction kicks in. Therefore we expect CBZ blood level to be lower at week 4 compared to week 1.

The formulation of CBZ that is FDA approved for bipolar mania is the ER capsule branded EQUETRO ($275) which may have slightly fewer side effects, e.g., less nausea. However, psychiatrists usually just prescribe generic IR carbamazepine ($30) and refer to the medication as Tegretol. If CBZ ER is desired, CARBATROL ER ($45) is exactly the same as Equetro, although FDA approved for seizures.

The advantage of CBZ over lithium and valproate is that CBZ does not cause weight gain or tremor. CBZ can be rather sedating, which can be desirable for acute mania.

CBZ may render birth control pills ineffective due to 3A4 induction. It is contraindicated during pregnancy. Teratogenic risks include "anticonvulsant face", neural tube defects, cleft palate, and malformations of the cardiovascular and urinary systems.

CBZ was recently found to be associated with stroke, whereas lithium and lamotrigine were not (Chen et al, 2019).

Dosing: The recommended dose for a manic episode is 400–600 mg BID, starting at 200 mg BID, and increasing by 200 mg/day. Starting at 200 mg TID would be reasonable for a hospitalized patient. Bipolar dosing is guided by clinical response, although most psychiatrists do check blood levels. When used for seizure disorders, the therapeutic CBZ blood level is 4–12 mcg/mL. For bipolar disorder, monitoring of blood levels may be useful for verification of drug compliance and assessing safety, but a therapeutic range is undefined. Remember, due to 3A4 auto-induction, CBZ levels will be lower at week 4 compared to week 1.

Dynamic interactions:
- Sedative/CNS depression (mild)
- Hyponatremia
- Serotonergic (weak)
- Hyperammonemia
- Decreases thyroid hormone
- Myelosuppression

Idiosyncratic interactions (unknown mechanism, rare):
- Neurotoxicity when combined with lithium
- Neurotoxicity when combined with verapamil (calcium channel blocker)

Kinetic interactions:
- "Shredder" in**D**ucer of several CYP enzymes
- UGT inDucer (lowers lamotrigine levels)
- P-glycoprotein in**D**ucer (increased removal of P-gp substrates from the brain), see page 9
- Increased metabolism of thyroid hormone
- 3A4 substrate

Carbamazepine **in<u>D</u>uces its own metabolism** (CYP3A4). The effect occurs within 2 to 3 weeks (**D**elayed), then stabilizes.

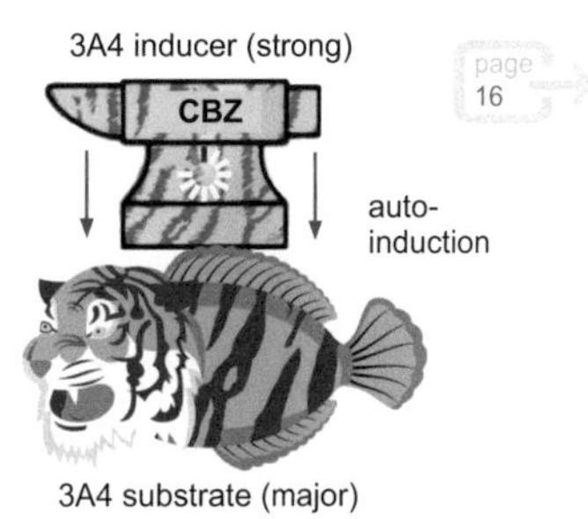

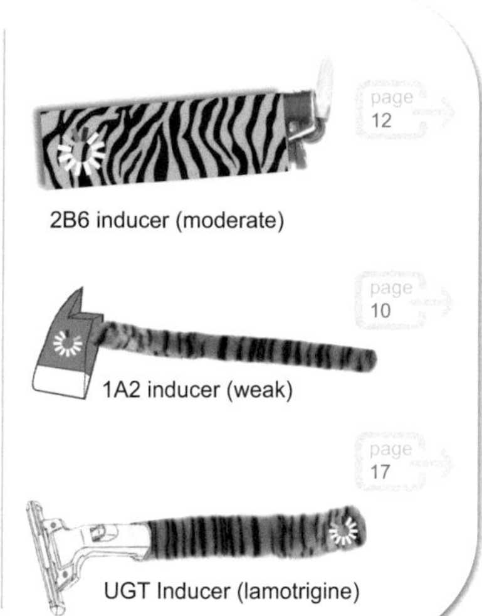

Continued...

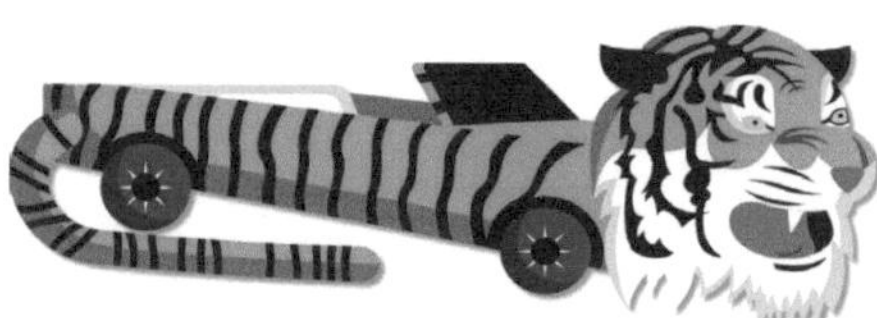

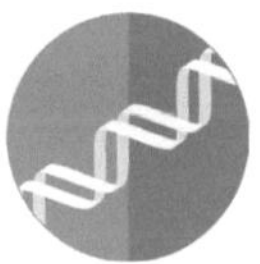

The FDA recommends Asian patients, who have a 10-fold higher incidence of CBZ-induced Stevens-Johnson syndrome (SJS) and toxic epidermal necrolysis (TEN), be screened for the **HLA-B*1502** allele, which would be a contraindication for starting CBZ.

Mnemonic: "Hey Look, Asian Blood! 1502, no Tegretol for you!"

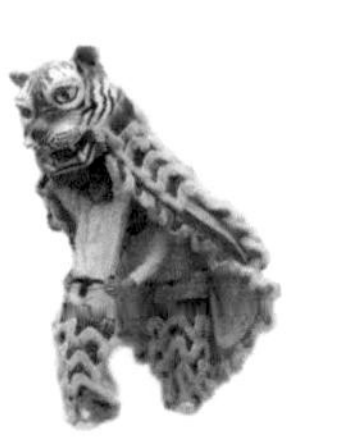

AEDs that are highly effective for **neuropathic pain**:

- Pregabalin (Lyrica)
- Gabapentin (Neurontin)
- Carbamazepine (Tegretol)

Pregabalin and gabapentin may cause weight gain, while carbamazepine does not.

Combinations with carbamazepine

Acute mania necessitates a combo of mood stabilizer + antipsychotic + benzodiazepine. Also, most individuals with bipolar I disorder are maintained on more than one medication. Since CBZ is a shredder inDucer, finding a suitable combination can be tricky.

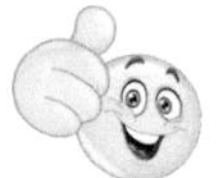

"Good" Combos - serum levels not significantly decreased by CBZ

- **Lithium** - although there have been rare cases of neurotoxicity with this combo, lithium ameliorates hyponatremia and neutropenia caused by CBZ.
- **Gabapentin** (Neurontin)
- **Fluphenazine** (Prolixin), even **long-acting injectable (LAI) Prolixin Decanoate**
- **Olanzapine** (Zyprexa)
- **Asenapine** (Saphris)
- **Loxapine** (Loxitane)
- **Iloperidone** (Fanapt
- **Ziprasidone** (Geodon)
- **The "LOT" benzodiazepines** (page 55) - **Lorazepam** (Ativan), **Oxazepam** (Serax), and **Temazepam** (Restoril)

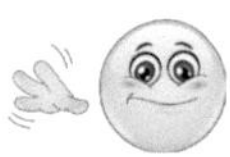

OK Combos - but higher doses will be needed

- **Lamotrigine** (Lamictal) - Use double dose; be vigilant for Stevens-Johnson syndrome (SJS).
- **Valproate** (Depakote) - Depakote is to be dosed based on VPA blood levels, as usual
- **Risperidone** (Risperdal) - **oral**—do not use long-acting injectable (LAI).
- **Haloperidol** (Haldol) - If using LAI Haldol Decanoate, consider supplementing with PO Haldol so that, if CBZ is stopped, the PO Haldol can be stopped also. Otherwise, serum haloperidol levels from the LAI will be too strong when induction is reversed.
- **Paliperidone** (Invega) - **oral**—do not use LAI
- **Aripiprazole** (Abilify) - **oral**—do not use LAI

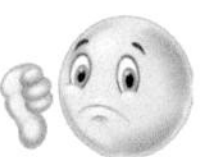

"Bad" Combos

- **Lurasidone** (Latuda) - contraindicated because lurasidone levels are Decimated by CBZ
- **Quetiapine** (Seroquel) - blood levels Decreased 5 -fold by CBZ; may need to use a higher quetiapine dose, which will be hazardous if CBZ is ever stopped (reversal of induction). If started along with CBZ for acute mania, quetiapine will work for a couple of weeks but by week 4 it will be essentially useless. This might not be a problem if mania is resolved and the prescriber and patient are aware of the interaction.
- **Clozapine** (Clozaril) - CBZ Decreases clozapine levels and both medications can suppress bone marrow.
- **Long-acting injectable (LAI)** formulations of aripiprazole, risperidone, or paliperidone

#244
2000
$9–$115

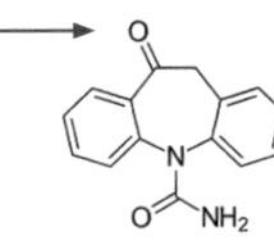

Oxcarbazepine (TRILEPTAL)

OX car baz a peen / tri LEP tal

"Oscar Leapt"

❖ Antiepileptic
❖ Voltage-gated sodium channel blocker
❖ Glutamate ⇩

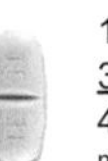

150
300
400
mg

Structurally, oxcarbazepine is the same as carbamazepine, other than this ketone.

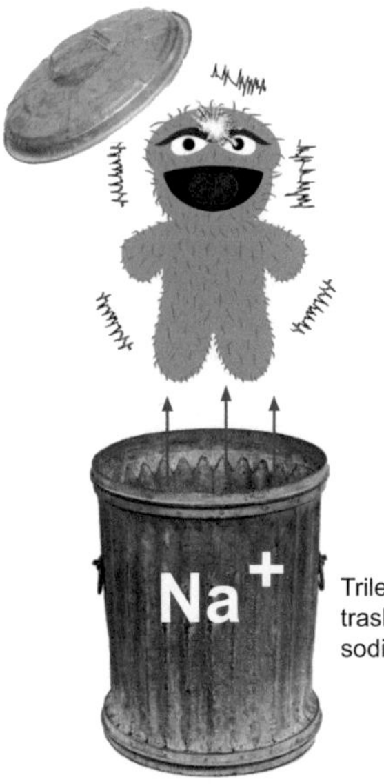

Signs of hyponatremia (sodium ≤ 130)

- ❖ Irritability
- ❖ Confusion
- ❖ Headache
- ❖ Blurred vision
- ❖ Weakness/fatigue
- ❖ Muscle cramps
- ❖ Nausea/vomiting

Risks with sodium ≤ 120

- ❖ Seizures
- ❖ Brain swelling
- ❖ Coma

Risk factors for hyponatremia:

- ❖ Polydipsia
- ❖ Sweating with sports
- ❖ Oxcarbazepine
- ❖ SSRI antidepressants
- ❖ Desmopressin (DDAVP)
- ❖ Diuretics

To decrease risk of hyponatremia during sports, drink Gatorade instead of water.

Dynamic interactions:
- ❖ Hyponatremia (major)
- ❖ Sedative (mild)
- ❖ Serotonergic (mild)

page 16

Kinetic interactions:
- ❖ Oxcarbazepine is a weak 3A4 inducer, unlikely to be of much clinical significance.

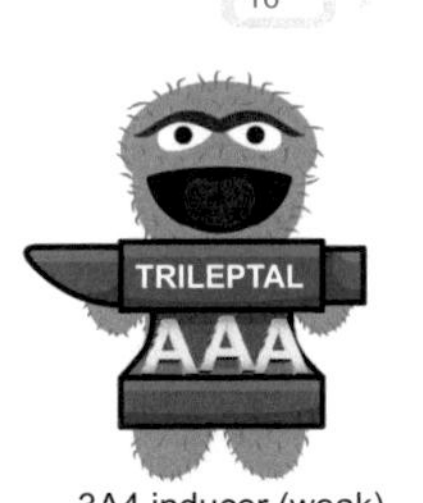

3A4 inducer (weak)

FDA-approved for:
- ❖ Focal seizures

Used off-label for:
- ❖ Bipolar disorder
- ❖ Trigeminal neuralgia

Oxcarbazepine (Trileptal) is FDA approved for seizure disorders and used off-label for bipolar disorder. Oxcarbazepine has several advantages over carbamazepine, but unfortunately there is less evidence for effectiveness of oxcarbazepine for bipolar disorder. It commonly causes hyponatremia, so it is necessary to monitor serum sodium with a metabolic panel (BMP or CMP). Normal sodium range is around 136–148. Symptoms of hyponatremia may occur at ≤ 130. Critical low sodium of ≤ 120 may cause seizures, brain swelling and coma. If hyponatremia is corrected too quickly, the myelin sheaths of nerve cells in the pons may be damaged by osmotic demyelination (central pontine myelinolysis).

	Carbamazepine (TEGRETOL)	Oxcarbazepine (TRILEPTAL)
Structure		
Entered U.S. market	1962	2000
Approx cost/30-day supply	$38	$20
FDA approved for	Seizure disorder Trigeminal neuralgia Bipolar I disorder (ER)	Focal seizures
Therapeutic drug monitoring	Required when used for seizure disorders. Traditionally checked when used for bipolar disorder.	May be useful, but not required.
Bipolar dosing	Start 200 mg BID. Target 400–600 mg BID or blood level 6–10 mcg/mL	Start 300 mg BID. Target 600–1200 mg BID
Risk of Stevens-Johnson syndrome (SJS)	Yes	Yes
HLA-B*1502 testing for Asians (SJS risk factor)	required	recommended
Risk of significant hyponatremia = Low sodium < 125 mmol/L	Yes, but less than with oxcarbazepine	Yes
Risk of bone marrow toxicity (Aplastic anemia, agranulocytosis)	Yes	minimal
Risk of hepatotoxicity	Yes	minimal
Inducer of drug metabolism	3A4 (strong) 2B6 (moderate) 1A2 (weak) UGT (lamotrigine)	3A4 (weak)
Auto-induction of own metabolism	Yes	No
Bioequivalent dosing for ER formulations	Yes (BID, same mg)	No (ER is weaker than IR)

This is So Dum!

Dosing: For off-label treatment of bipolar disorder, the author usually starts 300 mg BID x 2 days, then 300 mg TID x 2 days, then to the target dose of 600 mg BID. Maximum total daily dose is 2,400 mg (1,200 mg BID). As for any antiepileptic drug, taper to discontinue. Extended- and immediate-release formulations are not interchangeable on a mg-for-mg basis. When converting from Trileptal IR to the ER formulation (Oxtellar XR), a higher dose may be required.

#11
1993
$11–$92

Gabapentin (NEURONTIN)

gab a PEN tin / nur RON tin

"Gabba pen tin" = "Neuron tin"

- ❖ Antiepileptic
- ❖ Voltage-gated calcium channel blocker
- ❖ Glutamate ⇩

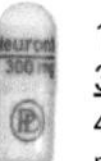

100
300
400
mg

FDA-approved for:

- ❖ Focal seizures
- ❖ Post-herpetic neuralgia
- ❖ Restless legs syndrome (as Horizant ER)

Used off-label for:

- ❖ Neuropathic pain
- ❖ Fibromyalgia
- ❖ Migraine prophylaxis
- ❖ Anxiety
- ❖ Bipolar disorder (adjunct)
- ❖ Alcoholism (sobriety maintenance)
- ❖ Alcohol withdrawal
- ❖ Cannabis use disorder
- ❖ Nightmares
- ❖ Improved quality of sleep

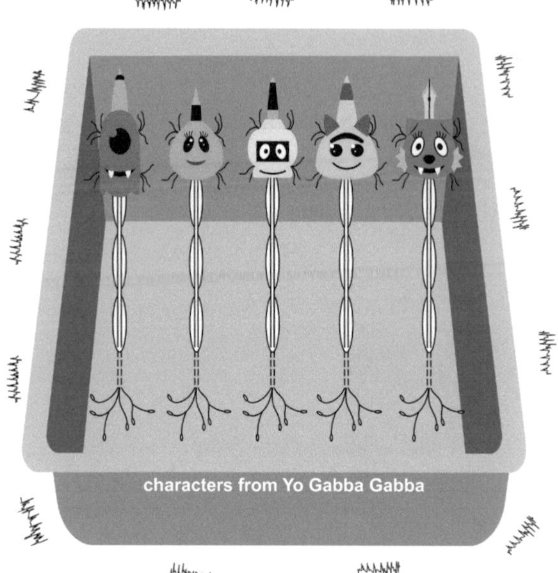

characters from Yo Gabba Gabba

Gabapentin (Neurontin) has the reputation of being a well-tolerated though not a particularly powerful antiepileptic drug (AED).

The name derives from its structural similarity to GABA, the brain's chief inhibitory neurotransmitter. Despite its name and structure, gabapentin does not affect GABA activity in any way. Gabapentin does not bind GABA receptors (as do benzodiazepines and barbiturates), inhibit GABA reuptake (like tiagabine), or block degradation of GABA (like vigabatrin). Gabapentin blocks voltage-gated calcium channels (as do lamotrigine, topiramate and pregabalin).

Gabapentin is the #1 prescribed medication of the AED class, and the #11 overall prescribed drug. Most commonly, gabapentin is prescribed for conditions other than seizure disorders, many of which are off-label. It is widely prescribed for neuropathic pain. Gabapentin is sometimes used adjunctively for bipolar disorder, but it has little, if any, mood stabilizing efficacy. It does have anxiolytic properties.

Gabapentin may cause modest weight gain. Some patients experience sedation, dizziness, ataxia, fatigue, and dyspepsia. There is a small risk of DRESS Syndrome (Drug Reaction with Eosinophilia and Systemic Symptoms), which is potentially fatal.

Neurontin is excreted unchanged in urine, making it immune from CYP interactions. There are no genetic polymorphisms that influence its metabolism. In other words, no one is a poor metabolizer or ultrarapid metabolizer of gabapentin.

As of 2020, gabapentin is not a DEA controlled substance. Some US states have begun regulating gabapentin, starting with Kentucky in 2017 as a result of gabapentin being detected in up to a third of the state's fatal overdoses. In 2020 the FDA required a label warning about the risk of life-threatening respiratory depression for patients with respiratory risk factors (COPD, the elderly, those taking opioids).

Gabapentin was initially regarded as having no abuse potential, but issues have arisen. Prison physicians no longer commonly prescribe it due to high rates of diversion. About 20% of individuals who abuse opioids will also overuse gabapentin because it can potentiate the opioid high. Otherwise, only 1–2% of patients overuse gabapentin.

Gabapentin is similar in structure and mechanism to pregabalin (Lyrica). Gabapentin and pregabalin constitute the gabapentinoid class of medication. Side effects attributed to pregabalin on the next page, such as peripheral edema, may also apply to gabapentin.

A gabapentin withdrawal syndrome is possible. It can include disorientation, anxiety, palpitations, diaphoresis, and abdominal cramps. Sudden withdrawal of any antiepileptic can precipitate a seizure, even for an individual without a seizure disorder.

Dosing: The lowest-strength capsule is 100 mg. The minimum effective dose is generally 300 mg TID. For seizure disorder, start 300 mg TID. For other conditions, the label recommends starting 300 mg QD x 1 day, then 300 mg BID x 1 day, then 300 mg TID. The maximum total daily dose is 3,600 mg, which is probably too high for psychiatric conditions. The author's target dose is 300–600 mg TID and occasionally as high as 900 mg TID. For patients with opioid use disorder, it is recommended not to exceed 900 mg daily (300 mg TID) due to risk of overdose (Gomes et al, 2017). For nightmares or improvement of sleep quality, a reasonable dose is 300–600 mg HS. As for any antiepileptic drug, taper to discontinue.

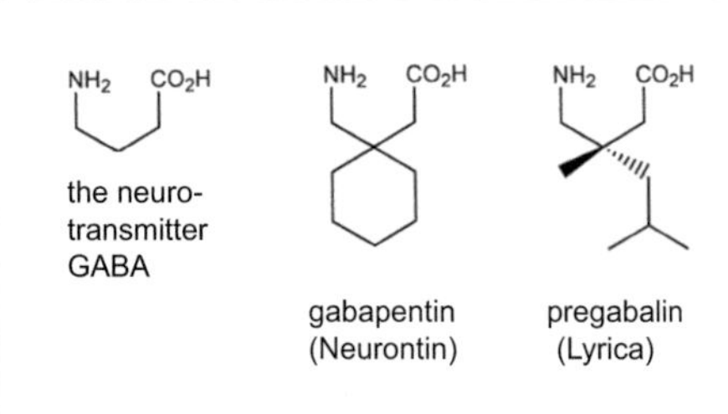

Dynamic interactions:

- ❖ Sedation/CNS depression (mild)
- ❖ Weight gain (modest)
- ❖ Respiratory depression

Kinetic interactions:

- ❖ None significant because it is excreted unmetabolized in urine - "in a bubble"

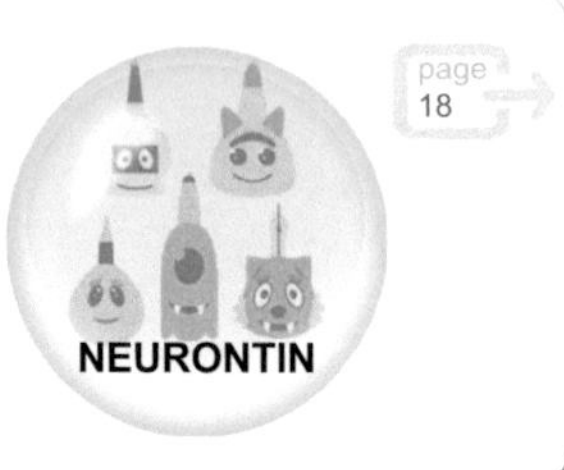

page 18

#83 (trending up)
2005
$18–$591

Pregabalin (LYRICA)

pre GAB a lin / LEER ik uh

"Preg gobblin' Lyrics"

- ❖ Antiepileptic
- ❖ Voltage-gated calcium channel blocker
- ❖ Glutamate ⇩
- ❖ DEA Schedule V

25, 50, 75, 100, 150, 200, 225 mg

FDA-approved for:
- ❖ Focal seizures (adjunct)
- ❖ Neuropathic pain
- ❖ Fibromyalgia
- ❖ Post-herpetic neuralgia

Used off-label for:
- ❖ Generalized anxiety
- ❖ Social anxiety
- ❖ Alcohol dependence
- ❖ Alcohol or benzo withdrawal

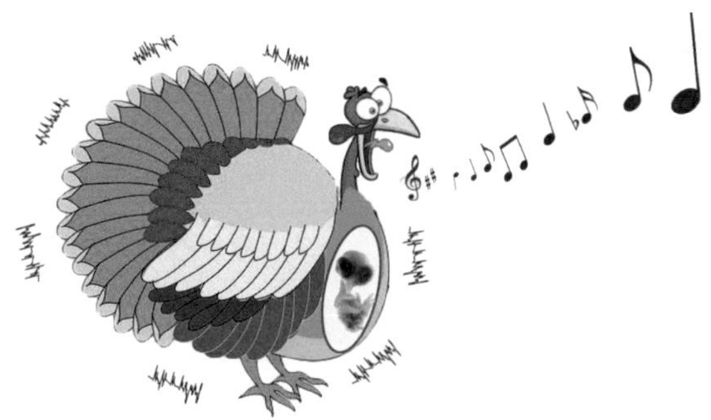

Pregabalin, FDA-approved in 2005, is a voltage-gated calcium channel blocker, as is gabapentin (Neurontin). Gabapentin and pregabalin constitute the gabapentinoid class of medication. Their structure is similar to GABA, but neither bind GABA receptors.

Lyrica is not metabolized, but rather excreted unchanged in the urine. Half-life is 6 hours, similar to that of Neurontin. Lyrica is a Schedule V controlled substance (least restrictive) because euphoria is possible. Generic pregabalin has been available since 2019.

It is approved for generalized anxiety in the UK. Large randomized-controlled trials supports its use (off-label) for generalized and social anxiety disorders.

Monographs in this book do not routinely address use during pregnancy, but since "preg" is in this drug's name—consider avoiding use of pregabalin during pregnancy. Teratogenicity is not expected, but pregabalin was not good for fetuses of animals given double the recommended human dose.

Side effects:
- ► Dizziness
- ► Sedation
- ► Headache
- ► Concentration problems
- ► Peripheral edema
- ► Weight gain (usually not)
- ► Angioedema (rare)
- ► Myoclonus (rare)
- ► Rhabdomyolysis (rare)

AEDs that are highly effective for **neuropathic pain**:

- ► Pregabalin (Lyrica)
- ► Gabapentin (Neurontin)
- ► Carbamazepine (Tegretol)

	Gabapentin (NEURONTIN)	Pregabalin (LYRICA)
Structure (similar to GABA)		
Entered U.S. market	1993	2005
Cost/30 days (January 2020)	$11/$92 (with/without GoodRx coupon)	$18/$591 (with/without GoodRx coupon)
FDA-approved for	Focal seizures; Restless legs syndrome; Post-herpetic neuralgia	Focal seizures (adjunct); Neuropathic pain; Fibromyalgia; Post-herpetic neuralgia
Mechanism	Voltage-gated calcium channel blocker	Voltage-gated calcium channel blocker
Metabolism	Excreted unchanged in urine	Excreted unchanged in urine
Usual dosing	TID	BID–TID
Controlled substance	Not federally, but is regulated in some states	Schedule V
Starting dose	300 mg QD x 1 day, 300 mg BID x 1 day, then 300 mg TID	50 mg TID, may incr. to 100 mg PO TID within 1 wk
Max dose	3,600 mg/day (1,200 mg TID) although this may be too much	600 mg/day (200 TID or 300 BID)

In 2020 the FDA issued a warning of respiratory depression in individuals with respiratory risk factors (COPD, obesity, those taking opioids). The warning applied to gabapentin also.

Dosing: For most indications, start 50 mg TID or 75 mg BID. May increase to total daily dose of 300 mg within one week; 300–600 mg/day in divided doses is an effective maintenance dose for generalized/social anxiety disorders; Maximum total daily dose is 600 mg.

Dynamic interactions:
- ❖ Sedation (mild)
- ❖ Respiratory depression

Kinetic interactions:
- ❖ None significant because it is excreted unmetabolized in urine - "in a bubble"

page 18

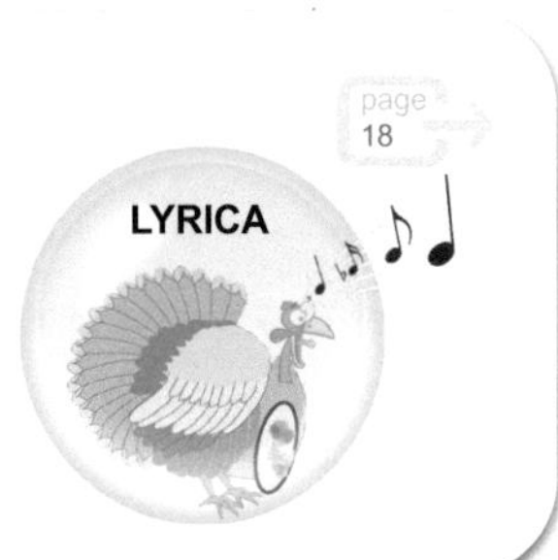

#85
1996
$4–$82

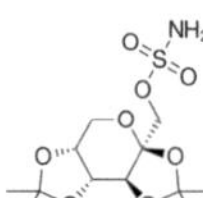

Topiramate (TOPAMAX)

toh PEER a mate / TOH pah max

"Top at max (speed on) Top (of) pyramid"

- Antiepileptic
- Voltage-gated sodium and calcium channel blocker
- Glutamate ⇩

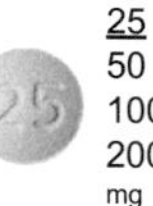

25
50
100
200
mg

FDA-approved for:

- Focal seizures
- Bilateral tonic-clonic seizures
- Lennox-Gastaut syndrome
- Migraine prophylaxis
- Obesity, long-term treatment (in combination with phentermine)

Used off-label for:

- Alcoholism (relapse prevention)
- Bipolar disorder (adjunct)
- Weight loss (monotherapy)
- Binge eating disorder
- PTSD
- Nightmares

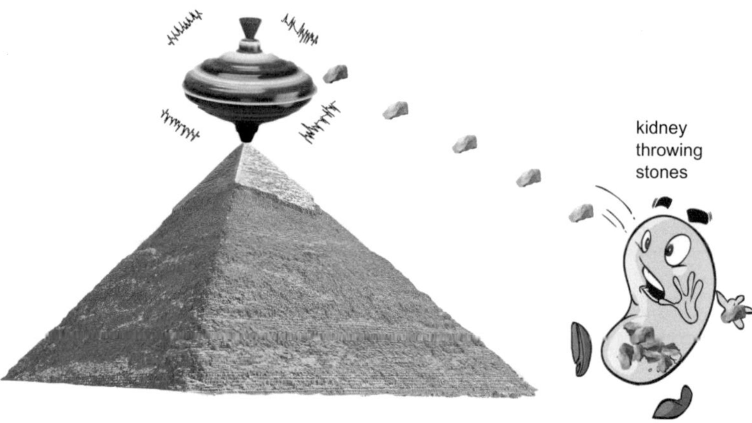

Topiramate is prescribed by psychiatrists for several off-label uses. The most compelling data is for preventing alcohol relapse. Although not FDA-approved for alcoholism, it is recommended in the 2015 US Veterans Affairs guidelines for moderate/severe alcohol use disorder.

Nicknamed "Dopamax" or "Stupamax", topiramate commonly causes cognitive problems including "brain fog", psychomotor slowing, difficulty concentrating and word-finding difficulty. Cognitive impairment due to topiramate is reversible, and usually only problematic at doses over 200 mg daily. A patient taking 200 mg BID told the author that, at a stoplight, she had trouble remembering if green meant stop or go. The recommended dose for epilepsy is 200–400 mg daily. It can be dosed lower for other purposes. The starting dose for any purpose, except nightmares, is 25 mg BID (25 mg HS for nightmares).

The two AEDs prescribed by psychiatrists that are highly effective for migraine prophylaxis are topiramate and valproate (Depakote, Depakene). The recommended topiramate dose to prevent migraines is 50 mg BID, which is not expected to impair cognition.

Paresthesia (tingling sensation) is common, and a favorable predictor of migraine prophylaxis. Dysgeusia (metallic taste) is possible.

Because topiramate is excreted unchanged in urine, there are few pharmacokinetic interactions. There are no genetic polymorphisms that affect its metabolism. In other words, no one is a poor metabolizer or ultrarapid metabolizer of topiramate.

Topiramate has undesirable carbonic anhydrase activity, hence alkalinizing urine and bringing a 15% risk of kidney stones with chronic use.

Another consequence of the carbonic anhydrase activity is lowered blood pH (acidification) due to raised urine pH (alkalization). Evidence of lowered blood pH is seen on a metabolic panel as low bicarbonate, which is listed as CO_2. Signs of metabolic acidosis (serum bicarbonate < 20 mmol/L) include tachycardia, headache, confusion, fatigue, nausea, and vomiting. Chronic acidosis can contribute to osteoporosis.

Topiramate is commonly prescribed off-label as an appetite suppressant. Topiramate ER is available in a fixed-dose combination with phentermine (appetite-suppressing stimulant) branded as Qsymia ($190) for long-term treatment of obesity. Qsymia is available only from certified pharmacies and certified prescribers to ensure female patients are counseled on the risk of birth defects. Topiramate itself increases the risk of oral clefts 4-fold.

Dosing: For nightmares, start 25 mg HS and go to 50 mg HS if necessary. For migraine prophylaxis or obesity, give 25 mg BID x 1 week then 50 mg BID. The maintenance dose for seizure disorders is 100–200 mg BID. Since topiramate impairs cognition when dosed 200 mg/day or higher, for other psychiatric uses try not to exceed 100 mg BID. For alcoholism titrate to 100 mg BID. Extended-release formulations of topiramate (Trokendi XR, Qudexy XR) can be dosed once daily.

Dynamic interactions:

- Sedation/CNS depression
- Increased risk of hyperammonemia with valproic acid (Depakene, Depakote), that can present as encephalopathy
- Increased risk of hypokalemia with hydrochlorothiazide (HCTZ)
- Increased risk of acidosis with metformin, which also decreases bicarb (CO2). Keep this in mind when prescribing weight loss medications. Metformin or topiramate can be prescribed off-label for weight loss, but they should not be prescribed in combination.

Topiramate is a weak 3A4 inDucer, which is insignificant at lower doses. However, if dosed > 200 mg/day, topiramate's induction of 3A4 may be clinically significant, i.e., by Decreasing blood levels of 3A4 substrates

page 16

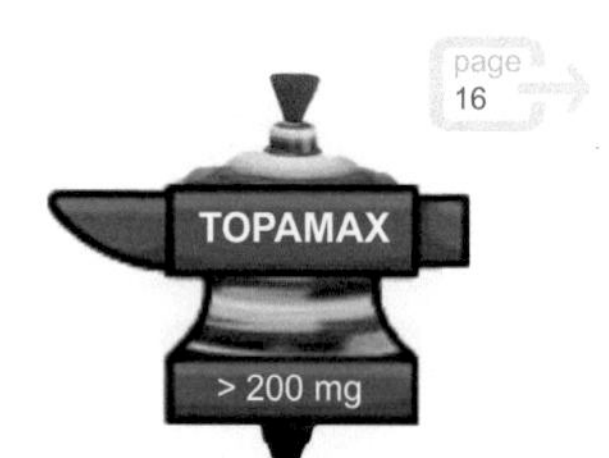

Topiramate can decrease lithium levels. As a carbonic anhydrase inhibitor, it raises urine pH, which increases excretion of lithium. The effect is expected to be mild and of little clinical significance. Topiramate can alter levels of other drugs whose excretion is affected by pH of urine.

page 26

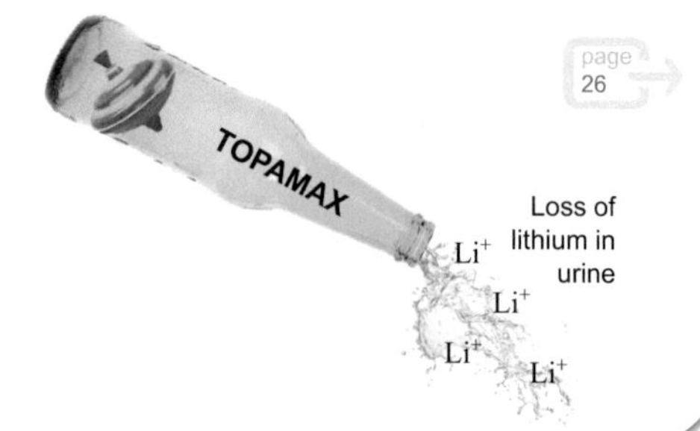

#89
2000
$6–$117

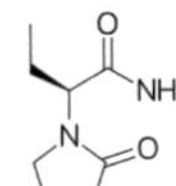

Levetiracetam (KEPPRA)

LEE ve tye RA se tam / KEP ruh

"Levitate Keeper"

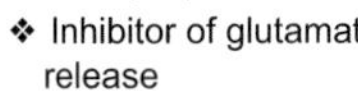

- ❖ Antiepileptic
- ❖ Inhibitor of glutamate release

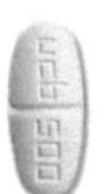

250
500
750
1000
mg

FDA-approved for:
- ❖ Focal seizures (adjunct)
- ❖ Juvenile myoclonic epilepsy (adjunct)
- ❖ Bilateral tonic-clonic seizures (adjunct)

Used off-label for:
- ❖ Other types of seizures

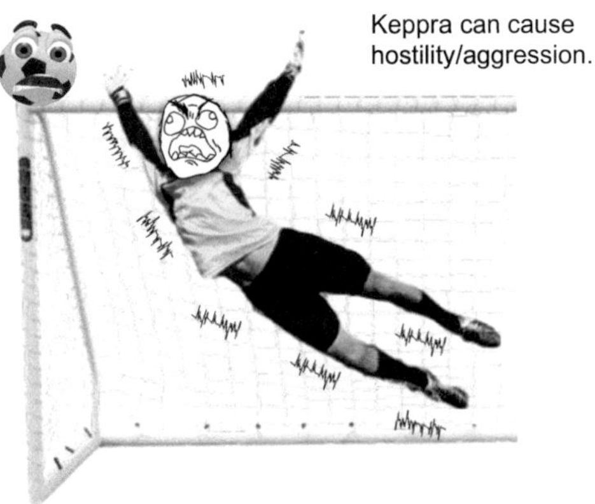

Keppra can cause hostility/aggression.

Levetiracetam entered the U.S. market in 2000 as an AED with a novel mechanism of action. It binds SV2A, a synaptic vesicle glycoprotein. This reduces the release of glutamate, the brain's principal excitatory neurotransmitter, thereby preventing hypersynchronization of epileptiform burst firing.

Levetiracetam has become one of the most prescribed medications for the treatment of epilepsy. It is not prescribed by psychiatrists. Advantages of levetiracetam as an AED include efficacy for a broad-spectrum of seizure types, lack of cognitive impairment, and lack of drug interactions. It can be started at an effective 500 mg BID dose on day one, which is also nice. Half-life is about 7 hours. 66% is excreted unchanged in the urine.

The most common side effects are dizziness, fatigue, and insomnia. The more troublesome problem with Keppra can be irritability and mood changes. This may occur to some degree in up to a third of patients taking the medicine (Dr. Robert Fisher, epilepsy.com). The array of psychiatric adverse effects may include depression, suicidal ideation, psychosis, hostility, and aggression. If a patient on Keppra experiences behavioral disturbance, they can be switched to brivaracetam (Briviact), a similar AED with a lower incidence of mood disruption.

Dosing: A typical adult dose for levetiracetam is 500–1500 mg twice a day. Dr. Fisher usually starts with 250 mg BID x 1 wk, then 500 mg BID x 1 wk, then 1000 mg AM + 500 mg PM x 1 wk, then 1000 mg BID. This is slower than the package insert suggests.

Alternate mascot: "Leave it to racist Kappers"

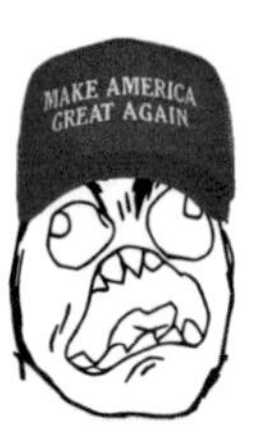

Dynamic interactions:
- ❖ Sedation (minimal)

Kinetic interactions:
- ❖ None significant
  - "in a bubble"

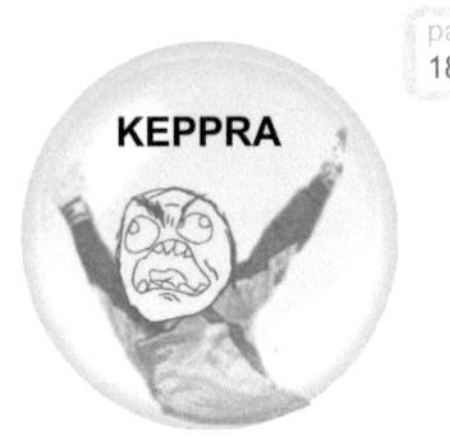

page 18

#201
1953
$21–$43

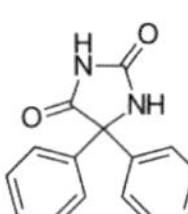

Phenytoin (DILANTIN)

fen i TOH in / di LAN tin

"Funny tunes Die laughin'"

- ❖ Antiepileptic
- ❖ Voltage-gated sodium channel blocker
- ❖ Glutamate ⇩

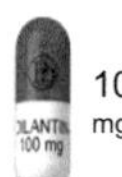

100 mg

FDA-approved for:
- ❖ Seizure disorder
- ❖ Status epilepticus
- ❖ Neurosurgery seizure prophylaxis

Used off-label for:
- ❖ Antiarrhythmic for suppression of ventricular tachycardia

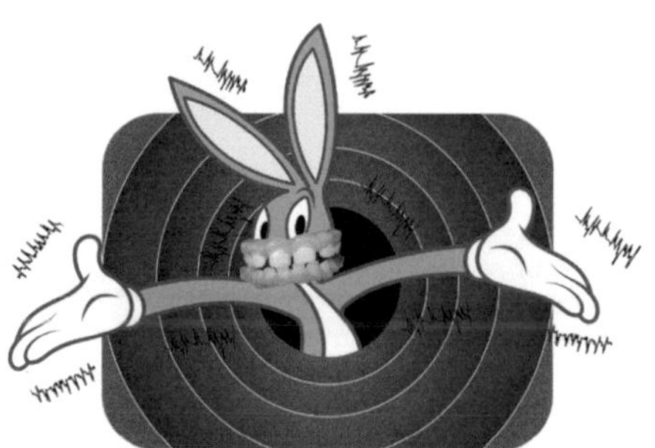

Phenytoin was FDA-approved as an antiepileptic in 1953. Phenytoin is not a first-line antiepileptic due to risks and side effects, and is not prescribed for psychiatric purposes.

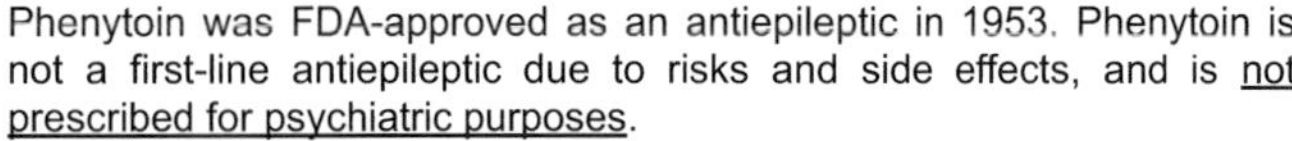

Phenytoin can literally make you ugly by increasing connective tissue growth factor (CTGF). Facial features may become coarse. About 50% of patients develop disfiguring gingival hypertrophy. Of all cases of drug-induced gingival overgrowth (DIGO), about 50% are attributed to phenytoin, 30% to cyclosporine (immunosuppressant for transplant recipients), and 10–20% to calcium channel blockers. Other possible consequences of increased CTGF are increased hair growth (arms, back, forehead) and Peyronie's disease (curved penis).

As with other antiepileptics, phenytoin can impair cognition and poses a risk of Stevens-Johnson syndrome (SJS).

Therapeutic index is narrow, so blood levels must be checked. Therapeutic serum range is 10 to 20 µg/mL, applicable to both antiepileptic and off-label antiarrhythmic uses. Nystagmus may be observed at levels greater than 20 µg/mL.

Dosing: For initial treatment of status epilepticus, give 15–20 mg/kg IV x 1. May give additional 10 mg/kg IV x 1 after 20 min if no response to initial dose. Begin maintenance dose 12 hours after the loading dose. For maintenance, aim for a trough blood level of 10–20 µg/mL, which may be achieved with 300–400 mg total daily dose divided BID or TID. Maximum per single dose is 400 mg. Note that phenytoin displays non-linear kinetics, i.e., doubling the dose will more than double the blood level.

The **"shredders"** are four **strong inDucers** of several CYPs, which cause countless chemicals to be quickly expelled from the body:

- ❖ **carbamazepine** (Tegretol) - antiepileptic
- ❖ **phenobarbital** (Luminal) - barbiturate
- ❖ **phenytoin** (Dilantin) - antiepileptic
- ❖ **rifampin** (Rifadin) - antimicrobial

Dr. Jonathan Heldt refers to the shredders as **"Carb & Barb"** in his book *Memorable Psychopharmacology*.

Dynamic interactions:
- ❖ Sedative

Kinetic interactions:
- ❖ "Shredder" inducer (see below)
- ❖ 2C9 substrate
- ❖ 2C19 substrate
- ❖ Increased metabolism of thyroid hormone

page 12

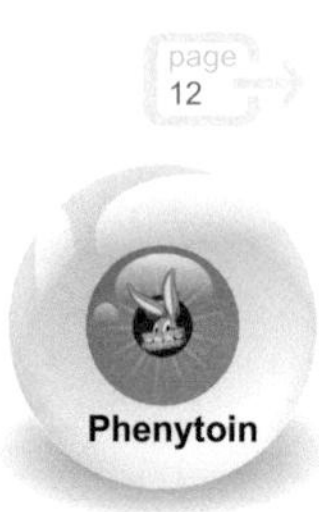

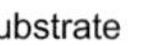

2C9 substrate

page 12

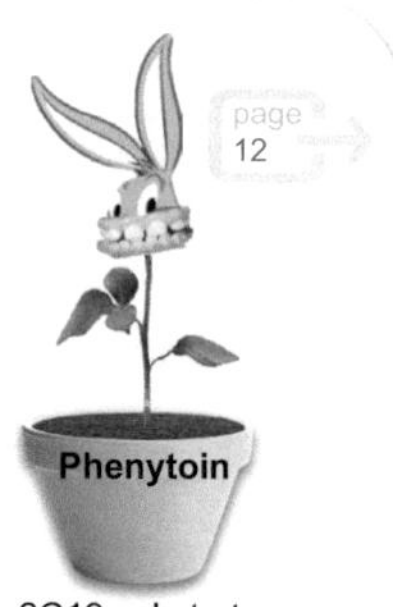

2C19 substrate

Phenytoin is a "shredder" of substrates of several CYP enzymes

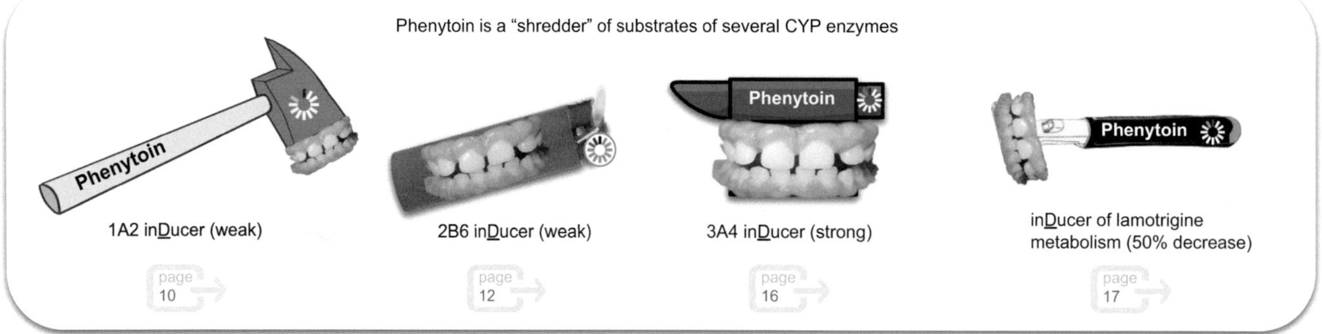

1A2 inDucer (weak) page 10

2B6 inDucer (weak) page 12

3A4 inDucer (strong) page 16

inDucer of lamotrigine metabolism (50% decrease) page 17

2000
$24–$188

Zonisamide (ZONEGRAN)

zoe NIS a mide / ZAHN uh gran

"Zone is mighty, Zone is grand"

- Antiepileptic
- Voltage-gated sodium channel blocker
- Glutamate ⇩

25
50
100
mg

FDA-approved for:
- Focal seizures

Used off-label for:
- Other types of seizures
- PTSD nightmares
- Sleep-related eating disorder
- Obesity
- Binge eating disorder
- Alcohol use disorder
- Migraine prophylaxis
- Parkinsonian symptoms associated with Lewy body dementia

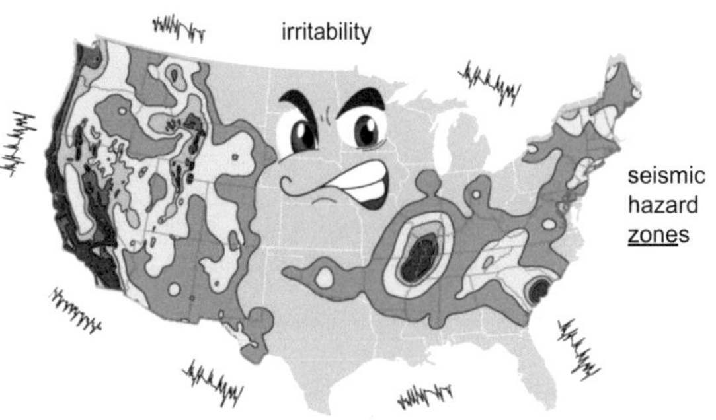

Zonisamide (Zonegran) is a broad-spectrum antiepileptic drug (AED) that blocks sodium and calcium channels and increases dopaminergic and serotonergic transmission. It is unrelated to other antiseizure medications.

Zonisamide decreases appetite and has been shown to decrease binge-eating. Cognitive impairment including "brain fog", confusion, difficulty concentrating, and word-finding difficulty are relatively common. It is not used as a mood stabilizer because it may cause irritability. There have been rare cases of zonisamide-induced psychosis.

Due to carbonic anhydrase inhibitor activity (although weak) there is a chance of kidney stones (4%) and metabolic acidosis. Aplastic anemia and agranulocytosis have been reported. Stevens-Johnson syndrome (SJS) and toxic epidermal necrolysis (TEN) have been reported. Oligohidrosis (decreased ability to sweat) has occurred with children.

Half-life is over 60 hours. About 30% is excreted unchanged in the urine.

Zonisamide has a sulfonamide structure, so it is contraindicated in patients allergic to sulfa drugs. Other sulfonamides include the antibiotic sulfamethoxazole (Bactrim, Septra) and the disease-modifying antirheumatic drug (DMARD) sulfasalazine. Unlike the other two sulfonamides, zonisamide does not have "sulfa" in its name.

Dosing: Start 100 mg daily. May increase by 100 mg q 2 weeks for a maximum of 600 mg. However, doses above 400 mg are rarely more effective. As with any antiepileptic medication, taper dose gradually to discontinue.

Zonisamide can cause weight loss.

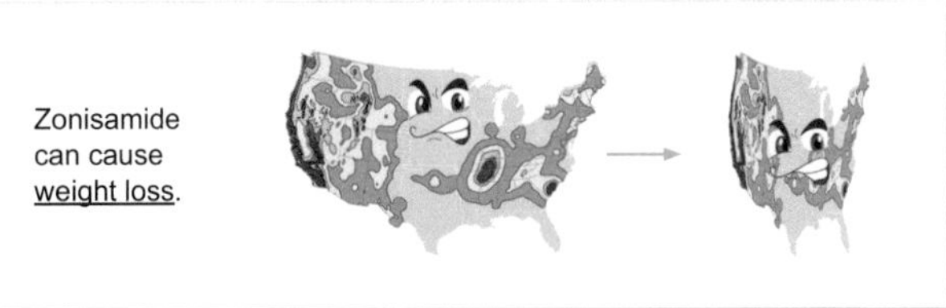

Dynamic interactions:
- Sedative (mild)
- Hypokalemia
- Metabolic acidosis
- Decreased renal perfusion

Kinetic interactions:
- Urine alkalization (minor)
- 3A4 substrate (minor)

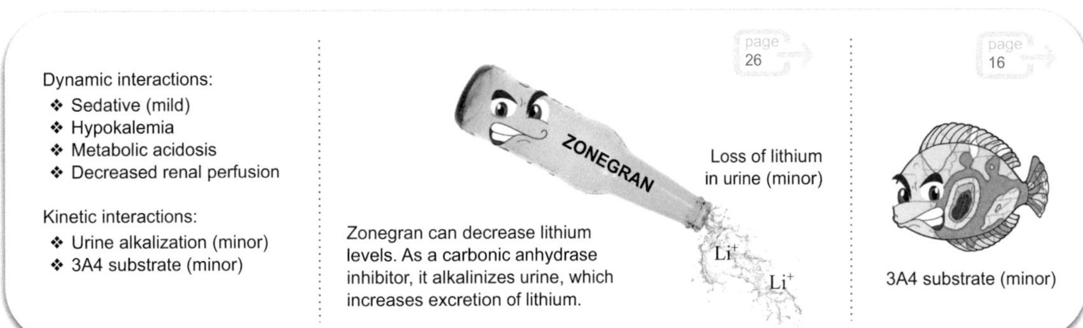

page 26

Loss of lithium in urine (minor)

Zonegran can decrease lithium levels. As a carbonic anhydrase inhibitor, it alkalinizes urine, which increases excretion of lithium.

page 16

3A4 substrate (minor)

2014
$858–$1,094

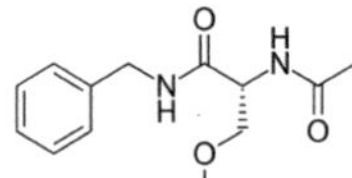

Lacosamide (VIMPAT)

la KOE sa mide / VIM pat

"Lacrosse Vampire"

- ❖ Antiepileptic
- ❖ Voltage-gated sodium channel blocker
- ❖ Glutamate ⇩
- ❖ DEA Schedule V

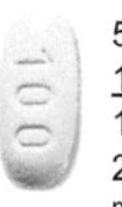

50
100
150
200
mg

FDA-approved for:

- ❖ Focal seizures, adjunct (2009)
- ❖ Focal seizures, monotherapy (2014)

Used off-label for:

- ❖ Other types of seizures

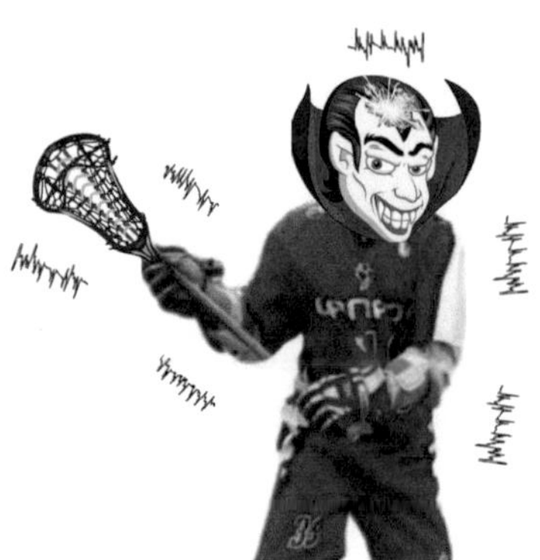

Lacosamide (Vimpat) is an antiepileptic synthesized from the amino acid serine. It blocks voltage-gated sodium channels, although in a different way than other antiepileptics.

Lacosamide is a Schedule V controlled substance (least restrictive) due to possible euphoria. It is not prescribed for psychiatric purposes although it has a low incidence of adverse psychiatric effects. As with any antiepileptic drug (AED), there is at least a slight risk of mood disruption. Labeling for all AEDs list suicidal thoughts as a possible risk.

Expect lacosamide to be an increasingly popular AED when it becomes available generically. The patent expires in 2022.

Side effects may include dizziness, headache, nausea, somnolence, fatigue, ataxia, diplopia, and tremor. Rarely, lacosamide causes first-degree AV block due to PR interval prolongation.

Dosing: For monotherapy of focal seizures, the maintenance dose is 150–200 BID; Start: 100 mg PO/IV BID, increase by 100 mg/day each week; FDA max is 400 mg/day; For conversion from AED monotherapy, give lacosamide maintenance dose for > 3 days before gradual withdrawal of previous AED over > 6 weeks; taper dose over > 1 week to stop.

page 18

Dynamic interactions:

- ❖ Use caution if combining with other PR interval prolonging drugs (e.g., beta blockers, calcium channel blockers).

Kinetic interactions:

- ❖ Minimal clinically significant kinetic interactions - "in a bubble"

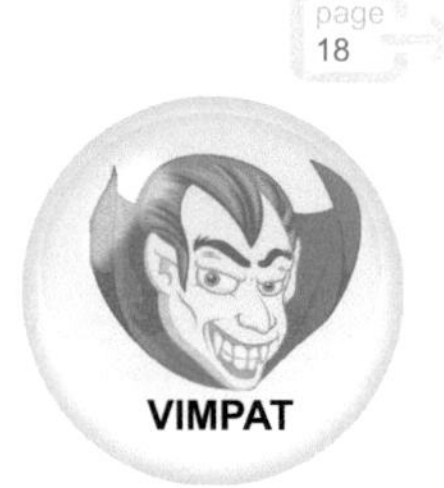

1960
$82–$253

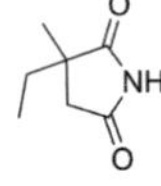

Ethosuximide (ZARONTIN)

ETH oh SUX i mide / zuh RON tin

"Zorro's Ethics suck!"

- ❖ Antiepileptic
- ❖ T-type calcium channel blocker

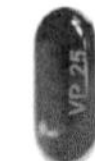

250
mg

FDA-approved for:

- ❖ Absence seizures

Used off-label for:

- ❖ N/A

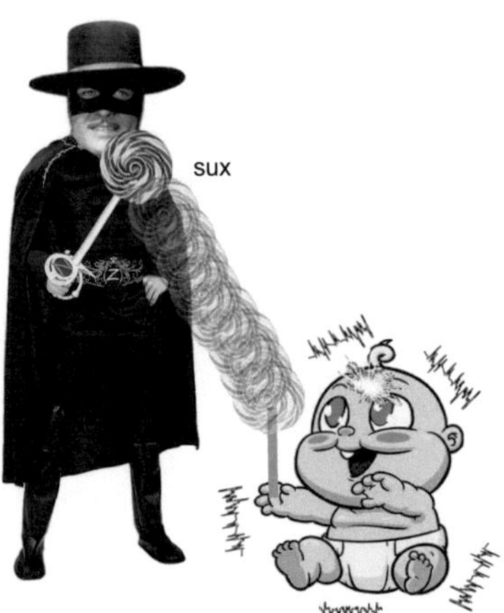

Child having petit mal seizure

Available since 1960, ethosuximide is the drug of choice for absence (petit mal) epilepsy. It is **in**effective for other seizure types. It seems to work by inhibiting low voltage-activated (T-type) calcium channels.

It is not used for psychiatric purposes and may rarely cause behavioral changes or even psychosis.

Other possible side effects include nausea, lethargy, headache and hiccups. Rare risks include hematologic abnormalities, erythema multiforme, Stevens-Johnson syndrome (SJS), and systemic lupus erythematosus (SLE).

Dosing: Maintenance dose for absence epilepsy is 250–750 mg BID; Start 250 mg BID, may increase by 250 mg/day q 4–7 days; Max is 1.5 g/day; The therapeutic serum range for ethosuximide is 40 to 100 mcg/mL; As with any AED, taper dose gradually to discontinue.

page 16

Dynamic interactions:

- ❖ Sedation/CNS depression

Kinetic interactions:

- ❖ 3A4 substrate

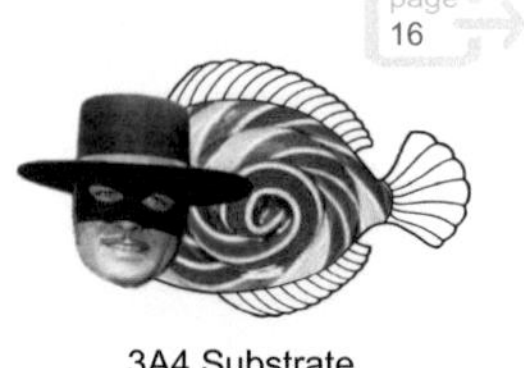

3A4 Substrate

Eslicarbazepine (APTIOM)

2013
$960–$1,182

ES li kar BAZ e peen / ap TEE om

"Slick car App time!"

❖ Antiepileptic
❖ Voltage-gated sodium channel blocker

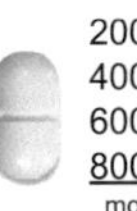

200
400
600
800
mg

FDA-approved for:
❖ Focal seizures, adjunct (2013)
❖ Focal seizures, monotherapy (2015)

Used off-label for:
❖ Other types of seizures

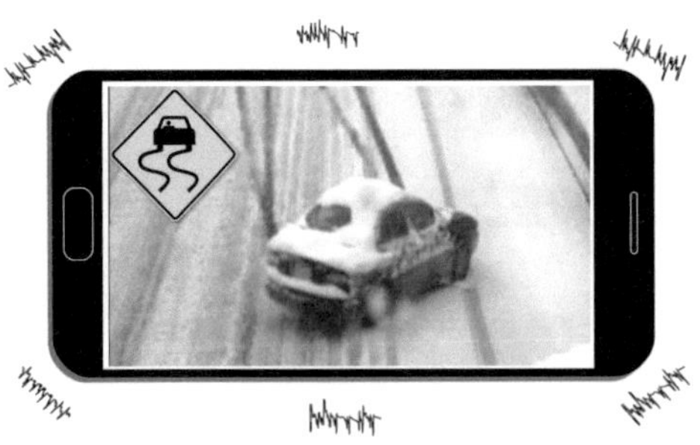

Eslicarbazepine is FDA-approved for treatment of focal seizures. It is not currently used as a mood stabilizer. It costs about $1,000 monthly and will not be off patent until 2021.

Eslicarbazepine is similar in structure and mechanism to carbamazepine (Tegretol, CBZ) and oxcarbazepine (Trileptal, OCBZ). Specifically, it is a prodrug of an active metabolite of oxcarbazepine.

Aptiom may have potential as a mood stabilizer, which is unsurprising given its similarity to CBZ. Nath et al (2012) reported successful treatment of a patient with bipolar mania who could not tolerate other anti-manic drugs.

Side effects can include dizziness, sedation, nausea, headache, diplopia, and ataxia. About 10% of patients stop it due to side effects. It is safer than CBZ, with similar risk profile to OCBZ. It is subject to more kinetic interactions than OCBZ but far fewer interactions than the shredder CBZ.

Patients who have experienced a serious rash from taking CBZ or OCBZ should avoid eslicarbazepine.

Dosing: Maintenance dose is 800–1600 mg QD; Start 400–800 mg QD, increase by 400–600 mg/day q week; Max is 1600 mg/day; As with any AED taper dose gradually to stop. Eslicarbazepine is 66% renally excreted, so the dose should be adjusted for those with renal impairment.

page 16

Dynamic interactions:
❖ Sedation/CNS depression
❖ Hyponatremia

Kinetic interactions:
❖ UGT substrate
❖ 3A4 inducer (minor)

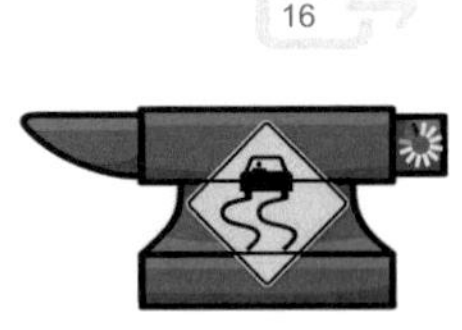

3A4 inducer (minor)

Rufinamide (BANZEL)

2009
$2,846–$3,494

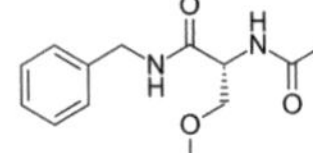

rue FIN a mide / BAN zel

"Ruffin' Ban"

❖ Antiepileptic
❖ Voltage-gated sodium channel blocker

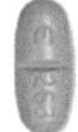

200
400
mg

FDA-approved for:
❖ Lennox-Gastaut syndrome (LGS)

Used off-label for:
❖ N/A

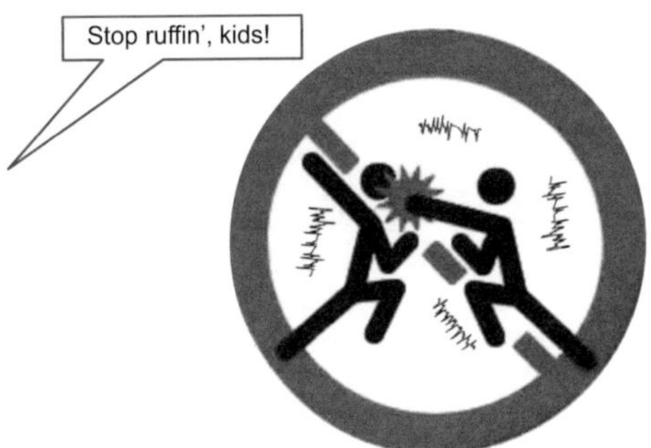

Lennox-Gastaut syndrome (LGS), pronounced *gas-TOE*, is a rare and severe form of childhood-onset epilepsy. LGS is characterized by multiple and concurrent seizure types, cognitive dysfunction, and slow spike waves on EEG. In 75% of cases there is an identifiable cause such as tuberous sclerosis, perinatal hypoxia or meningitis.

Rufinamide was released in 2009. It is FDA-approved for LGS in children ≥ 4 years old. Rufinamide works by prolonging the inactive state of voltage-gated sodium channels, thus stabilizing the neuronal membranes. It costs about $3,000 monthly, but a generic form may be available sometime after 2022.

Rufinamide shortens QT interval, which does not pose a clinical risk, unless patients have familial short QT syndrome or in combination with other QT shortening meds such as lamotrigine (Lamictal), digoxin, or magnesium. Contrast this with the many psychiatric medications that prolong QT.

Dosing: Start: 200–400 mg BID, increase by 400–800 mg/day every 2 days to 1600 mg BID which is both the recommended maintenance dose and FDA max; It should be given with food to promote absorption. If not taken with food, serum levels will be decreased up to 50%; Taper dose by 25% every other day to stop.

page 16

Dynamic interactions:
❖ Sedation/CNS depression

Kinetic interactions:
❖ UGT substrate
❖ Rufinamide is a minor CYP3A4 inDucer, unlikely to be of any clinical significance other than in combination with triazolam (Halcion), which rufinamide decreases by 35%.

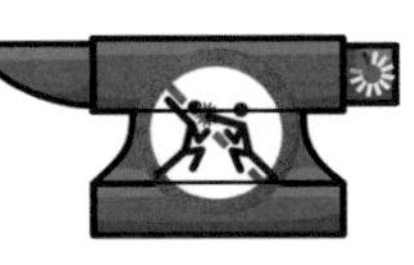

3A4 inducer (minor)

1993
$138–$438

Felbamate (FELBATOL)

FEL ba mate / FEL bah tol

"Fell bat / Fell bam!"

- ❖ Antiepileptic
  - ⇧ GABA activity
  - ⇩ Glutamate activity

400
600
mg

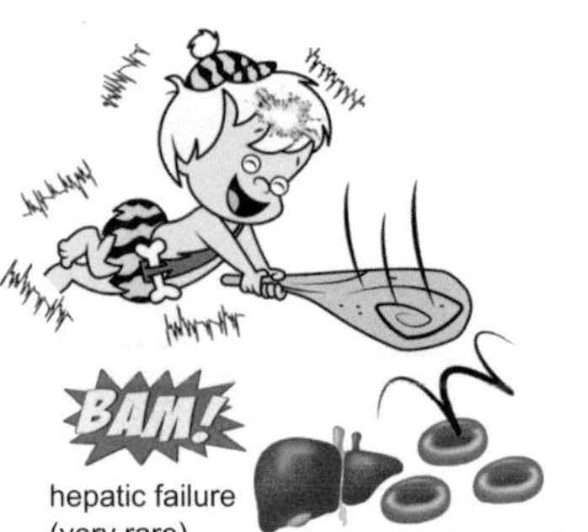

hepatic failure (very rare)

aplastic anemia (very rare)

FDA-approved for:

- ❖ Seizure disorders refractory to other antiepileptics

Felbamate (Felbatol), approved in 1993, is the first antiepileptic with dual actions on excitatory (NMDA) and inhibitory (GABA) activity in the brain. Specifically, felbamate inhibits NMDA responses and strengthens GABA responses. This unique combination of effects could account for its broad spectrum of antiepileptic activity (Rho JM et al, 1994). Although structurally similar to the anxiolytic meprobamate (Miltown, Schedule IV), felbamate is not a controlled substance.

In 1994, one year after its release, the FDA placed a warning on the label about risk of aplastic anemia and hepatic failure. A registry was created, but was discontinued after more than 1,000 patients had been entered and no adverse events were reported (Sofia et al, 2000). It is not to be used as a first-line medication, and the patient must sign an informed consent form acknowledging the risks. Felbamate is not available in Canada, the UK, or Australia.

Compared to other antiepileptics, felbamate is less likely to cause psychiatric adverse events or impair cognitive functioning. However, it is not prescribed by psychiatrists.

Felbamate is structurally similar to meprobamate (Miltown), the "minor tranquilizer" which became the first blockbuster psychotropic drug in the 1950s as an (abusable) anxiolytic.

page 194

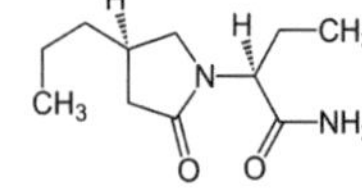

meprobamate

Dynamic interactions:

- ❖ Sedation/CNS depression
- ❖ Antiplatelet effects

Kinetic interactions:

- ❖ Felbamate decreases plasma concentrations of carbamazepine (Tegretol) by about 30% but increases concentrations of the active metabolite carbamazepine-10,11-epoxide by about 60% (Howard JR et al, 1992).
- ❖ Felbamate increases levels of phenytoin (Dilantin) and valproate (Depakote).

page 14

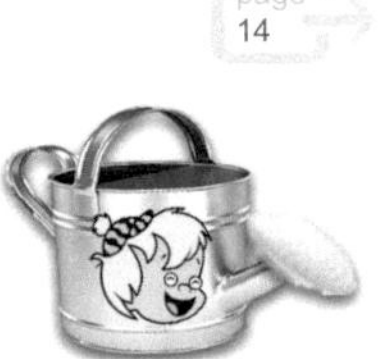

2C19 inHibitor (moderate)

page 16

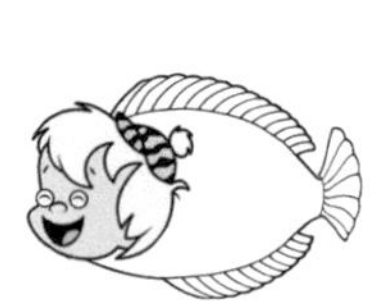

3A4 Substrate (major)

2016
$1,134–$1,390

Brivaracetam (BRIVIACT)

BRIV a RA se tam / BRIV ee act

"Brave act (in a) Brave race"

- ❖ Antiepileptic
- ❖ Inhibitor of glutamate release
- ❖ DEA Schedule V

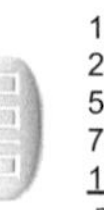

10
25
50
75
100
mg

FDA-approved for:

- ❖ Focal seizures

Used off-label for:

- ❖ Temporal lobe epilepsy
- ❖ Focal impaired awareness seizures
- ❖ Focal aware seizures
- ❖ Secondarily generalized seizures

Brivaracetam (Briviact) was approved in 2016 for adjunctive treatment of focal seizures in patients ≥ 16 years old. New drugs for epilepsy are often approved only as adjunctive treatment for focal seizures, because researchers aren't going to do placebo-controlled trials as monotherapy for individuals with generalized seizures. Once approved, new antiepileptic are typically used for several types of refractory seizures off-label. As expected for a new drug, it costs over $1,000 monthly.

Brivaracetam is an analog of levetiracetam (Keppra). As with levetiracetam, brivaracetam may cause anxiety and depression, and can be associated with aggression and psychosis. Psychiatric adverse reactions were reported in 13% of patients receiving brivaracetam (compared to 8% for placebo). Disturbance of mood and behavior is less severe than with levetiracetam. The main side effects of brivaracetam are somnolence and sedation (16%). It is a Schedule V (five) controlled substance (least restrictive schedule).

Brivaracetam has no off-label uses beyond seizure control. Psychiatrists do not prescribe it.

Unlike some antiepileptics, brivaracetam has a clearly defined mechanism of action. It binds selectively to synaptic vesicle protein 2A (SV2A) in the brain. Brivaracetam has a more rapid onset of action than levetiracetam and about a 20-fold higher affinity for SV2A than levetiracetam. Brivaracetam is also a partial antagonist on neuronal voltage-gated sodium channels.

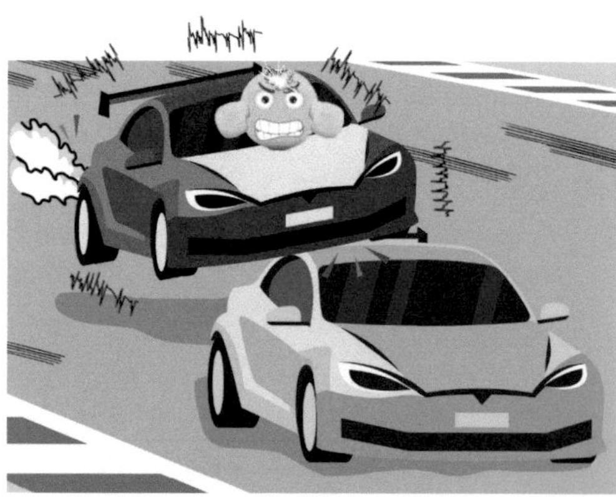

Brivaracetam may cause aggression (but less so than levetiracetam)

Dynamic interactions:

- ❖ Sedation/CNS depression

Kinetic interactions:

- ❖ Rifampin (moderate 2C19 inDucer) Decreases brivaracetam levels by almost half.
- ❖ 2C19 poor metabolizers have about 40% higher brivaracetam levels.

page 14

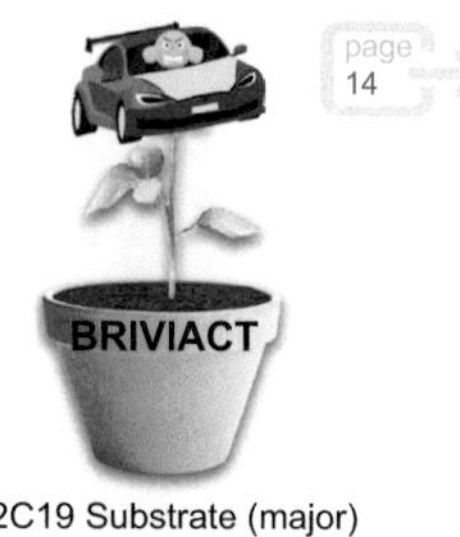

2C19 Substrate (major)

1998
$66–$226

Tiagabine (Gabitril)

ti AG a bean / GAB ih tril

"Tiger beans (on the) GABA trail"

❖ Antiepileptic
❖ GABA reuptake inhibitor

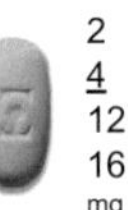

2
4
12
16
mg

FDA-approved for:

❖ Focal seizures, adjunct

Used off-label for:

❖ Focal seizures, monotherapy
❖ Other seizure types
❖ Anxiety disorders
❖ Neuropathic pain
❖ Sleep quality

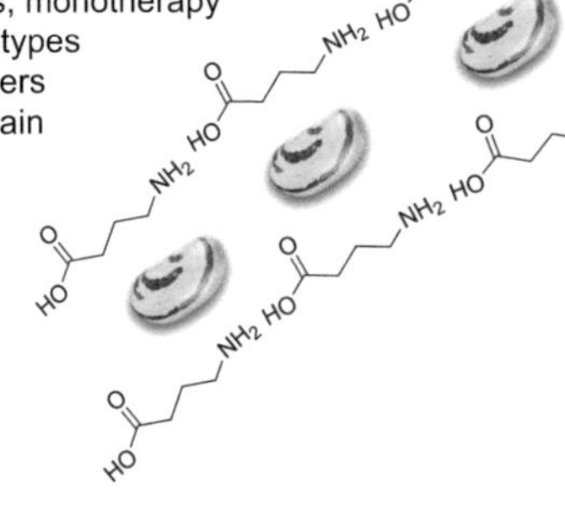

Tiagabine (Gabitril), released in 1998, is a specific GABA reuptake inhibitor, doing so by blocking GABA Transporter 1 (GAT-1). Currently, it is the only available medication with this mechanism of action.

It has been used off-label to increase deep sleep (stage 3 and 4, slow wave) to make a person feel more rested in the morning.

The main side effect is dizziness, followed by somnolence. Less common side effects include syncope, tremor, paresthesia and memory difficulties. Tiagabine can interfere with color perception, which was demonstrated in 41% of patients (Sorri et al, 2005).

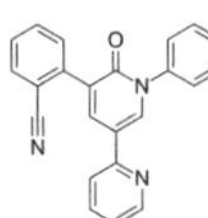

The evidence supporting tiagabine for psychiatric purposes is very weak, and its use for mood or anxiety is discouraged. Tiagabine may *induce* seizures in those without epilepsy, particularly if combined with medications that lower seizure threshold. It can cause status epilepticus in overdose situations.

Dosing: For focal seizures, the maintenance dose is 32–56 mg/day divided BID–QID; Start 4 mg QD x 1 week, then 4 mg BID x 1 week, then may increase by 4–8 mg/day q week; Max is 56 mg/day; Take with food; As with any AED taper dose gradually to stop.

page 16

Dynamic interactions:

❖ Sedation/CNS depression

Kinetic interactions:

❖ 3A4 substrate (major) - When combined with a 3A4 inducer, the half-life of tiagabine is reduced (from 8 hours) to about 5 hours.

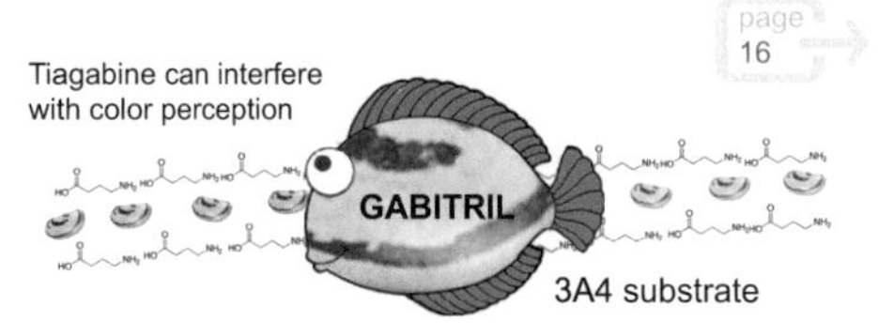

2014
$485–$1,161

Perampanel (FYCOMPA)

per AM pa nel / fye COM puh

"FICO Perm panel"

❖ Antiepileptic
⇧GABA activity
⇩ Glutamate activity
❖ DEA Schedule III

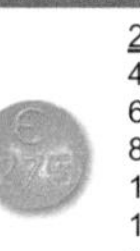

2
4
6
8
10
12
mg

FDA-approved for:

❖ Adjunctive treatment of focal seizures and tonic-clonic seizures in patients ≥ 12 years

Used for:

❖ Temporal lobe epilepsy
❖ Focal impaired awareness seizures
❖ Focal aware seizures
❖ Secondarily generalized seizures
❖ Tonic-clonic seizures

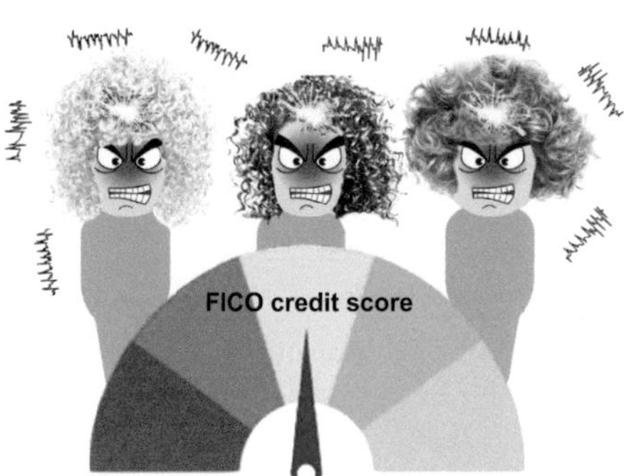

Perampanel (Fycompa) was approved in 2014 as a first-in-class noncompetitive AMPA receptor antagonist. AMPA receptors are a subtype of glutamate receptors involved in excitatory neuronal activity.

Perampanel carries a **black box warning** for severe psychiatric and behavioral reactions that can be serious or life-threatening, particularly hostility and aggression. Alternate mnemonics include "Fight-compa" and "Fight complicator".

Fycompa is a Schedule III controlled substance due to potential to induce euphoria. Very high doses produce dissociation similar to ketamine, although less pleasant.

Dose-dependent side effects include dizziness, somnolence, and blurred vision. Perampanel is not recommended for those with severe hepatic or renal impairment.

page 16

Dynamic interactions:

❖ Sedation/CNS depression

Kinetic interactions:

❖ 3A4 substrate (major) - Blood levels of perampanel are decreased 67% by carbamazepine (Tegretol) and 50% by phenytoin (Dilantin).

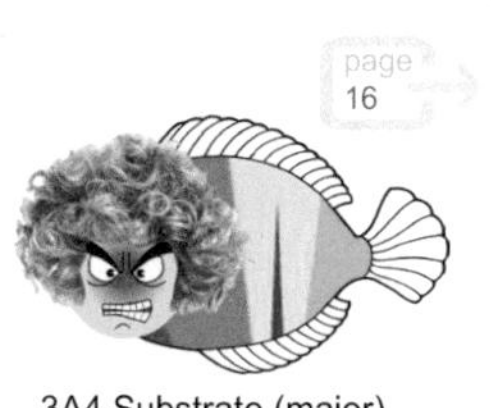

3A4 Substrate (major)

2020
$975–$1,010

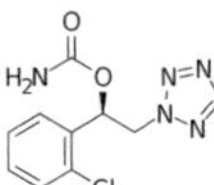

Cenobamate (XCOPRI)

sen oh BAM ate / EX cop ree

"Cinnabon Ex-couple"

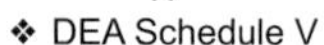

- ❖ Antiepileptic
- ❖ $GABA_A$ modulator
- ❖ DEA Schedule V

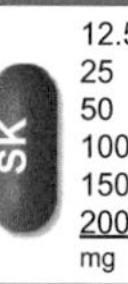

FDA-approved for:
- ❖ Partial-onset seizures (adults)

Cenobamate (Xcopri) is the newest antiepileptic drug (AED), released in 2020. There are some serious risks, side effects and kinetic drug-drug interactions.

Dosing is similar to lamotrigine (Lamictal), with a slow titration to a recommended dose of 200 mg over 11 weeks. As with lamotrigine, maximum dose is 400 mg—but titration of lamotrigine only takes 5 weeks. The slow titration of cenobamate is necessary to avoid Drug Reaction with Eosinophilia and Systemic Symptoms (DRESS), also known as multiorgan hypersensitivity. There were no cases of DRESS among over 1,000 patients with adherence to the slow titration schedule.

Cenobamate shortens QT interval and is contraindicated with Familial Short QT Syndrome. QTc interval under 300 is dangerous.

Dose-dependent side effects are common (36% at 200 mg; 57% at 400 mg) including somnolence/fatigue, dizziness, diplopia/blurred vision, cognitive impairment, and headaches. Dropout rates were 11%, 9%, and 21% respectively for patients randomized to receive Cenobamate 100 mg/day, 200 mg/day, and 400 mg/day (versus 4% for placebo).

Cenobamate is a Schedule V (five) controlled substance (least restrictive) due to the possibility of euphoric feelings at high doses. The risk of psychiatric adverse effects appears to be about 1 in 333. All antiepileptics have a risk of suicidal ideation. In the clinical trial there were 4 suicides among over 25,000 patients, versus none for 16,000 patients on placebo. Causation was not established. A withdrawal syndrome was observed with sudden discontinuation, including tremor, mood disturbance, and insomnia.

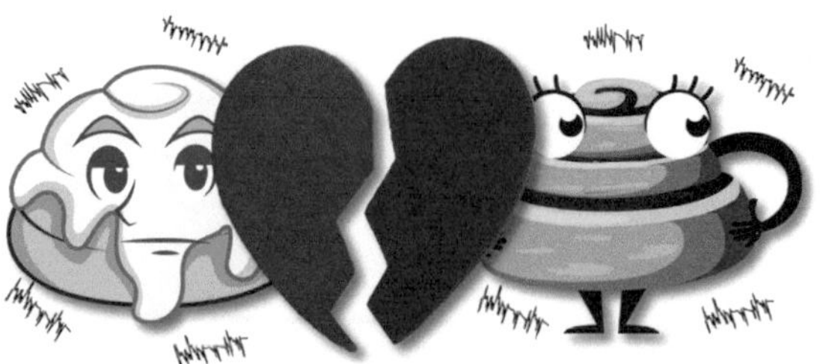

At 400 mg (maximum dose), liver enzymes were elevated with ALT greater than 3x upper limit of normal in almost 3% of patients. Cenobamate may also elevate serum potassium.

Dosing: The initial dose is 12.5 mg QD, to be titrated over 11 weeks to the recommended maintenance dose of 200 mg QD; May take with or without food, at any (consistent) time of day; The recommended titration schedule should not be exceeded to avoid DRESS; Maximum dose is 400 mg QD (200 if mild/moderate hepatic impairment); To discontinue, taper over at least 2 weeks.

Dynamic interactions:
- ❖ Sedation/CNS depression
- ❖ QT shortening
- ❖ Hypokalemia
- ❖ Liver enzyme elevation

Kinetic interactions:
- ❖ 2C19 in**H**ibitor
  - Increases levels of phenytoin (Dilantin) by 75%, requiring dose adjustment
  - Increases levels of phenobarbital (Luminal) and active metabolite of clobazam (Onfi)
- ❖ 3A4 in**D**ucer
  - Decreases levels of hormonal contraceptives and carbamazepine (Tegretol)
- ❖ UGT in**D**ucer
  - Decreases levels of lamotrigine (Lamictal)

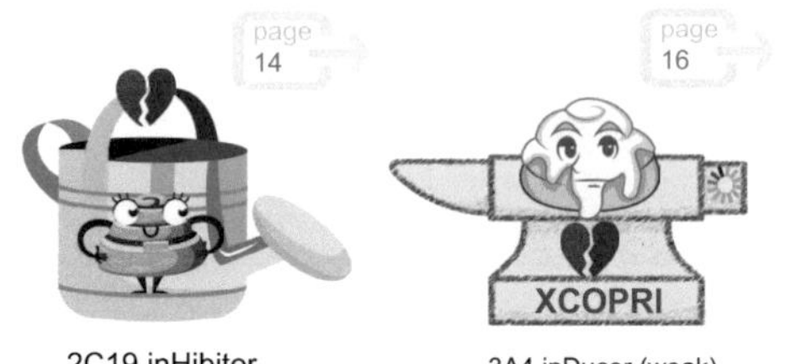

page 14
2C19 inHibitor

page 16
3A4 inDucer (weak)

2009
$3,772–$10,670

HO, NH2, O — gamma-vinyl-GABA (GVG)

Vigabatrin (SABRIL)

vi GAB a trin / SAB reel

"Violent GABA Sabre!"

- ❖ Antiepileptic
- ❖ GABA transaminase inhibitor

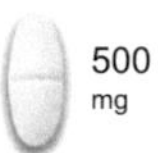

500 mg

FDA-approved for:

- ❖ Focal impaired awareness seizures in adults who are refractory to several antiepileptic drugs
- ❖ Monotherapy for infantile spasms

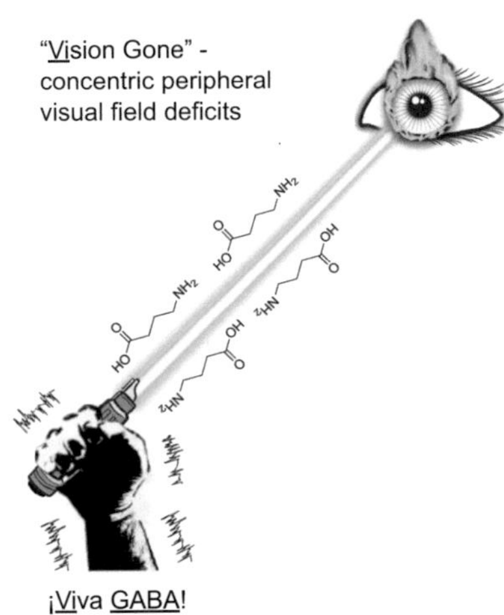

"Vision Gone" - concentric peripheral visual field deficits

¡Viva GABA!

Vigabatrin, also known as GVG (gamma-vinyl-GABA), was approved in 2009. It is a first-line treatment for infantile spasms (West syndrome) particularly when associated with tuberous sclerosis.

The "Vi" stands for vinyl, but it could be for "vision gone" due to risk of irreversible retinal damage. GVG is available through a restricted distribution program which includes exams for peripheral visual field deficits. Concentric peripheral visual field deficits are common with vigabatrin. For patients over age 12, 40% have visual loss at > 6 months of treatment. Visual loss is less common for younger patients. Affected individuals may not notice the peripheral visual loss until they are left with tunnel vision.

GVG has been available in other countries for many years. It is incredibly expensive in the US.

Vigabatrin increases concentration of GABA in the CNS by inhibiting GABA transaminase, an enzyme that degrades GABA. An alternate mnemonic is ¡Viva GABA!

About 20% of children < 3 years old treated with vigabatrin will have MRI evidence of white matter edema in the brain. This is reversible and may not "matter" clinically. It does not appear to occur in individuals ≥ 3 years old.

Other adverse effects may include weight gain, balance problems, somnolence, violent behavior, depression, suicidal ideation and expressive language disorder.

Dosing: Maintenance dose is 1,500 mg BID; Start 500 mg BID; May increase by 500 mg/day in weekly intervals; As with any AED, taper to stop.

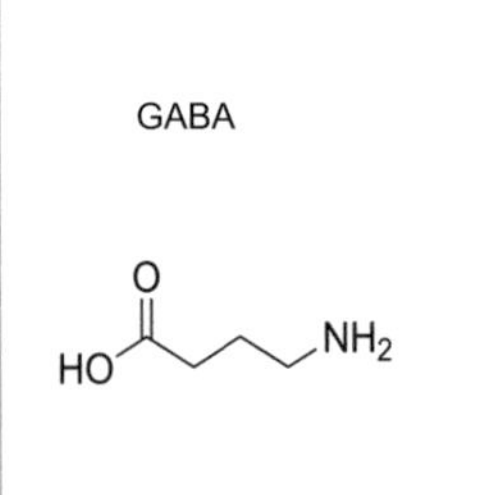

page 18

Dynamic interactions:

- ❖ Sedation/CNS depression

Kinetic interactions:

- ❖ Vigabatrin is renally eliminated, with no significant kinetic interactions - "in a bubble"

SABRIL

This Venn Diagram serves as an introduction to our next medication, cannabidiol (CBD).

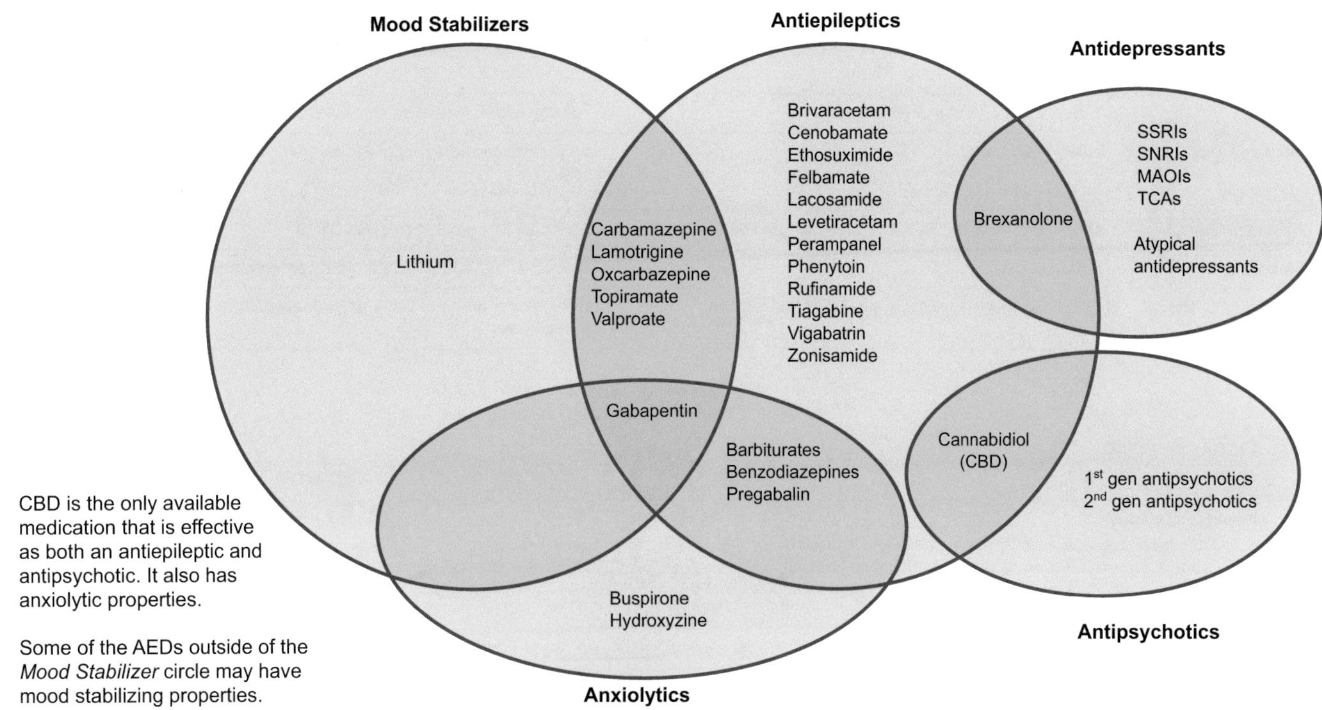

CBD is the only available medication that is effective as both an antiepileptic and antipsychotic. It also has anxiolytic properties.

Some of the AEDs outside of the *Mood Stabilizer* circle may have mood stabilizing properties.

2018
$1,290–$3,041

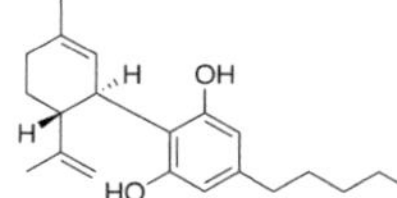

Cannabidiol (CBD; EPIDIOLEX)

can na bi DI ol / e pid e oh LEX

"Cannabis B.I.D. oil"

- ❖ Cannabinoid
- ❖ Antiepileptic
- ❖ Antipsychotic
- ❖ Neuroprotectant
- ❖ Non-controlled

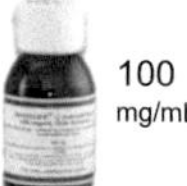

100 mg/mL

FDA-approved for:
- ❖ Lennox-Gastaut syndrome
- ❖ Dravet syndrome

Used off-label for:
- ❖ Schizophrenia
- ❖ Anxiety

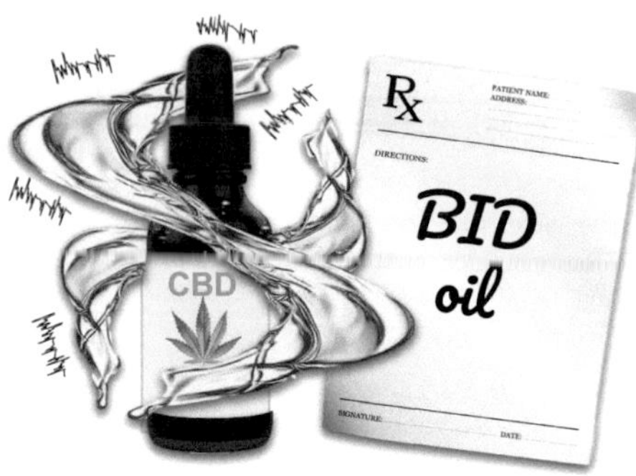

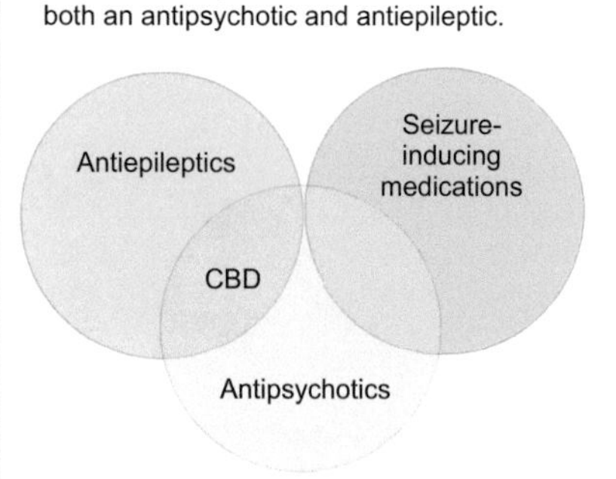

Epidiolex, pharmaceutical grade cannabidiol (CBD), was FDA-approved in 2018 for treatment of seizures associated with Lennox-Gastaut syndrome (LGS) and Dravet syndrome in children (age 2 and older). Lennox-Gastaut syndrome (LGS) is a type of childhood-onset epilepsy starting between 2–6 years of age. LGS is characterized by a triad of multiple seizure types, intellectual impairment, and characteristic EEG findings.

CBD is one of over 100 cannabinoids contained in marijuana. It should not be confused with "medical marijuana". In 2018 the DEA labeled Epidiolex as having low potential for abuse, classifying it as a Schedule V (five) controlled substance (lowest level of restriction). In 2020 the DEA dropped the restriction, so Epidiolex is no longer a controlled substance.

In clinical trials for schizophrenia, the subjects themselves were unable to tell whether they were in the treatment or placebo group.

CBD is an indirect antagonist of CB1 and CB2 cannabinoid receptors. CBD is an antipsychotic, neuroprotectant, and appetite suppressant which does not get the consumer "high". In many ways it is the opposite of tetrahydrocannabinol (THC), the main psychoactive component of cannabis. THC is a CB1 and CB2 agonist which makes it "The High Causer" in marijuana. Pure CBD is **not likely to cause a false positive drug screen** for marijuana (THC).

Epidiolex is an oral solution that (thankfully for the purpose of this mnemonic) is dosed BID. Somnolence is the main side effect of CBD. It has a good safety profile, but hepatotoxicity is possible.

CBD appears to work as an antiepileptic by inactivating voltage-gated sodium channels of the neuronal cell membrane.

CBD has demonstrated efficacy for schizophrenia at high dose. It is postulated to work as an antipsychotic through the endocannabinoid system. It is not FDA-approved for schizophrenia, but the future is promising. CBD may also be effective for social anxiety (Blessing EM et al, 2015).

Over-the-counter CBD oil is legal in all 50 states as long as it is extracted from the hemp plant, a variety of cannabis containing minimal THC. Of 84 online products tested, only 30% contained the advertised amount of CBD, and 21% contained THC (Boon-MIller et al, 2017).

Dosing: The dose for schizophrenia is 800–1,200 mg daily, which is at least $1,000 of the OTC product monthly. For anxiety, 25–200 mg daily is a reasonable dose. Reputable CBD products include Elixinol, Encore Life and Bluebird Botanicals.

	Tetrahydrocannabinol (THC)	Cannabidiol (CBD)
Pure Rx form	Dronabinol (Marinol), nabilone (Cesamet) - Schedule III	Epidiolex
Psychoactive?	The High Causer in marijuana; cognitive impairment	No "high" feelings, but may reduce anxiety
Psychosis	Cannabis use in adolescence triples the risk of psychotic disorders (Jones HJ et al, 2018)	Antipsychotic properties
Seizure	Epileptogenic (lowers seizure threshold)	Anticonvulsive (raises seizure threshold)
Neurotoxicity	Likely neurotoxic	Likely neuroprotective (antioxidant and cholinergic)
Munchies?	Yes. The Hunger Causer.	No; May cause weight loss.
FDA approval	Dronabinol (Marinol) to stimulate appetite (1985)	Epidiolex for pediatric seizures (2018)
Mechanism	CB1 and CB2 agonist	Indirect antagonist of CB1 and CB2 receptors
Drug interactions	Pure THC has few clinically significant interactions	Substrate of 3A4 and 2C19. InHibitor of 2C9, 2C19, UGT enzymes and others.

Dynamic interactions:
- ❖ Sedation/CNS depression

Kinetic interactions:
- ❖ 2C19 inHibitor (strong) - CBD may increase levels of 2C19 substrates such as diazepam (Valium) and clobazam (Onfi). Clobazam, a benzodiazepine approved for Lennox-Gastaut syndrome, is increased 3-fold by CBD.
- ❖ CYP3A4 substrate (minor)
- ❖ UGT inhibitor

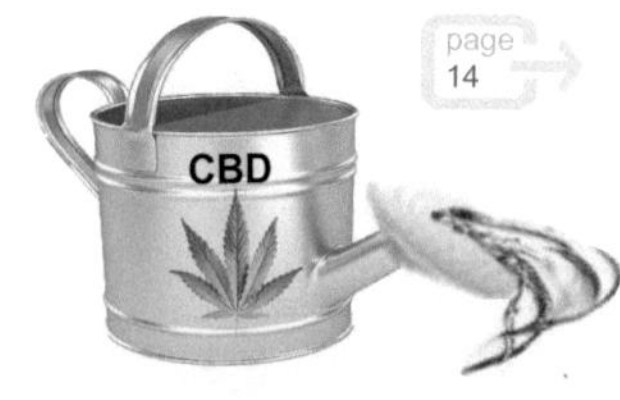

page 14

2C19 inHibitor (strong)

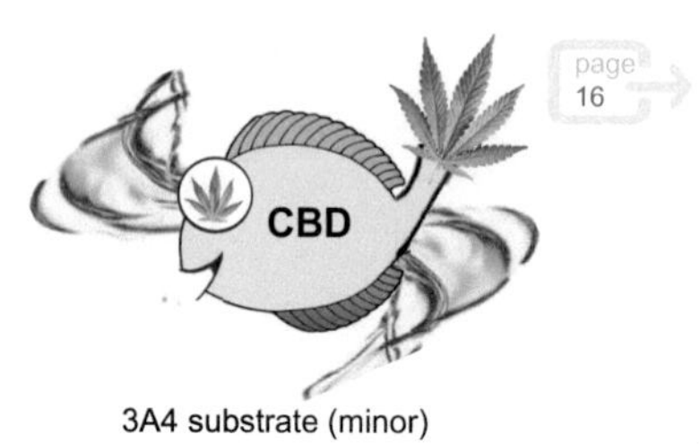

page 16

3A4 substrate (minor)

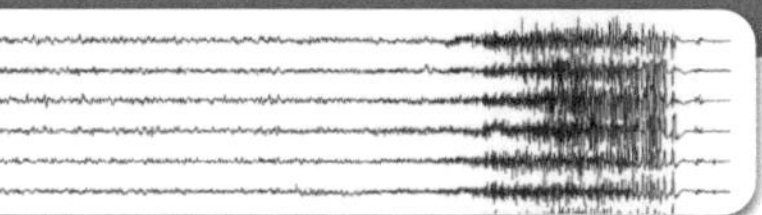

Epileptogenic Drugs

Medications that lower seizure threshold

Seizure threshold is the minimum electrical shock necessary to induce a seizure, as could be measured with electroconvulsive therapy (ECT). Antiepileptic drugs (AEDs) raise seizure threshold. Epileptogenic drugs decrease seizure threshold, thereby increasing the likelihood of a spontaneous seizure. Seizures due to epileptogenic medications tend to occur early in treatment or when dose is increased. Be careful when combining seizure-threshold-lowering medications due to aggregate risk of convulsions. "Convulsants" (see below) are agents that were given for the purpose of causing seizures, historically.

Class	Epileptogenic medications	Medications with minimal to no risk of seizures
Antipsychotics	#1 Clozapine (Clozaril) 10x risk at high dose #2 Olanzapine (Zyprexa) 3x #3 Quetiapine (Seroquel) 2x #4 Chlorpromazine (Thorazine) 2x	Risk is minimal for other antipsychotics. The following appear to be especially safe: risperidone, haloperidol, fluphenazine, thiothixene and some rarely used FGAs (molindone, pimozide, thioridazine). The only antipsychotic with antiepileptic activity is cannabidiol.
Antidepressants	#1 Maprotiline (Ludiomil) TCA, very high risk #2 Amoxapine (Asendin) TCA, high risk #3 Clomipramine (Anafranil) TCA 1–3% risk #4 Bupropion IR* (Wellbutrin) 1–2% risk—minimal with SR or XL None of these are commonly prescribed. *Most Wellbutrin prescriptions are SR or XL formulations.	For a long time, there has been a misconception that all antidepressant drugs have proconvulsant effects (Kanner, 2016). Many antidepressants do cause seizures with overdose, but excluding tricyclics and bupropion IR, the risk of seizure with antidepressants at a therapeutic dose is less than placebo, actually cutting risk of seizure in half (Alper et al, 2007). Note that depression itself lowers seizure threshold. MAOIs have the lowest seizure risk. Bupropion extended-release formulations (Wellbutrin SR and XL) at standard doses have minimal seizure risk.
Mood stabilizers	Lithium	All other mood stabilizers are antiepileptic drugs.
Anxiolytics	Buspirone (Buspar)	Benzodiazepines are antiepileptics. Beware of withdrawal seizures from any seizure-threshold-lowering medication. Alprazolam (Xanax) has a particularly high risk of withdrawal seizures due to short half-life.
Flumazenil	Flumazenil (Romazicon), the antidote for BZD overdose, is an antagonist at the BZD binding site on the GABA(A) receptor. For a brain accustomed to benzos, the addition of flumazenil is very likely to precipitate a seizure.	Since the body does not produce endogenous BZDs, flumazenil has no effect when administered in the absence of a BZD.
ADHD medications	Atomoxetine (Strattera) Methylphenidate (Ritalin, Concerta, etc) Amphetamine (Dexedrine, Adderall, Vyvanse, etc)	The antihypertensives used for ADHD: - Clonidine (Catapres) - Guanfacine (Tenex, Intuniv)
Antihistamines/ Anticholinergics	Trihexyphenidyl (Artane) Diphenhydramine (Benadryl) - in overdose or withdrawal Hydroxyzine (Vistaril) - in overdose or withdrawal	N/A
Cognitive enhancers	Donepezil (Aricept) Rivastigmine (Exelon) Memantine (Namenda)	N/A
Narcolepsy meds	Sodium oxybate (Xyrem) - sedative Modafinil (Provigil) - stimulant	N/A
Muscle relaxants (antispasmodics)	Baclofen (Lioresal) - GABA(B) agonist - in overdose Cyclobenzaprine (Flexeril) - tricyclic Methocarbamol (Robaxin)	Tizanidine (Zanaflex) - alpha-2 agonist Orphenadrine (Norflex) Carisoprodol (Soma)
Pain medications	Tramadol (Ultram) Tapentadol (Nucynta) Opioids (most)	Acetaminophen (Tylenol) NSAIDs
Other	Caffeine Cocaine Ginkgo biloba (herbal) Ondansetron (Zofran) - antiemetic PDE inhibitors (Viagra, etc)	Acetazolamide (Diamox) is a diuretic with many uses including glaucoma, intracranial hypertension, and altitude sickness. It is FDA-approved for seizure disorders but tolerance to the antiepileptic effect develops within weeks. It has value in treatment of epilepsy when taken for 14 day periods with one week's stop in between (Hoddevik, 2000).

Withdrawal seizures may be produced by abrupt discontinuation of any medication that raises seizure threshold, especially those with short half-lives. Withdrawal-induced seizures are seen with antiepileptic drugs, benzodiazepines (especially alprazolam), barbiturates, alcohol, anaesthetics, baclofen, carisoprodol (Soma), 1st gen antihistamines (diphenhydramine, hydroxyzine), and doxepin (TCA).

Historical convulsant	Trivia
Pentetrazol	GABA(A) receptor blocker, initially used as a circulatory and respiratory stimulant. Starting in 1934 it was used in high doses for shock therapy, i.e., intentionally producing convulsions in the treatment of depression. Because of uncontrollable seizures, it was replaced by electroconvulsive therapy (ECT), which debuted in 1938. The FDA revoked approval for pentetrazol in 1982.
Flurothyl	GABA(A) antagonist, used experimentally (by inhalation) for shock therapy in 1953 as an alternative to ECT. Flurothyl induced seizures were deemed clinically equal to electrical seizures with lesser effects on cognition and memory. Nonetheless, flurothyl is no longer used for shock therapy.

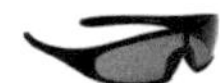

100% blue-light-blocking glasses (orange-tinted) were found highly effective for treatment of acute mania, adjunctively to standard antimanic medications (Henriksen et al, 2016). Patients hospitalized for mania were instructed to wear their glasses from 6pm to 8am, other than when lights were out.

The control group wore gray-tinted lenses. All subjects were managed with medications as usual. Results were dramatic, with improvement seen within 3 days. The blue blocking glasses group ended up requiring substantially fewer sedating medications (hypnotics, anxiolytics, antipsychotics) than those randomized to the control group. The mechanism likely involves the suprachiasmatic nucleus of the hypothalamus, where melatonin also acts. The glasses used in the study are available from Lowbluelights.com.

The original approach started in the 1990s as (actual, not virtual) darkness therapy. This involved keeping the manic patient in pitch darkness from 6pm to 8am.

Blue is the shortest wavelength of light on the visible spectrum. The retina contains melanopsin photoreceptors that only detect blue light, projecting to the suprachiasmatic nucleus (SCN), which is the brain's "master clock" in the hypothalamus. When these receptors are not exposed to blue light, the master clock thinks it is immersed in total darkness. Melatonin also signals to the SCN that it is dark, by binding MT1 and MT2 melatonin receptors.

For individuals with bipolar disorder, a strategy to prevent mania would involve wearing the glasses for 1–2 hours before bedtime (The Carlat Psychiatry Report, February 2019). Note the incidence of mania peaks in the spring when the amount of sunlight rapidly increases (Parker et al, 2018), typically in April.

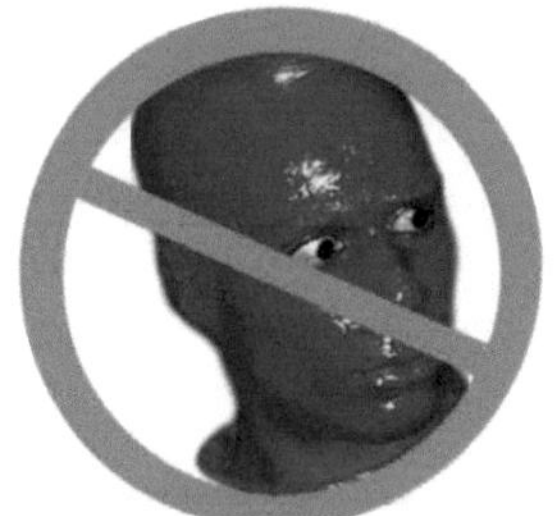

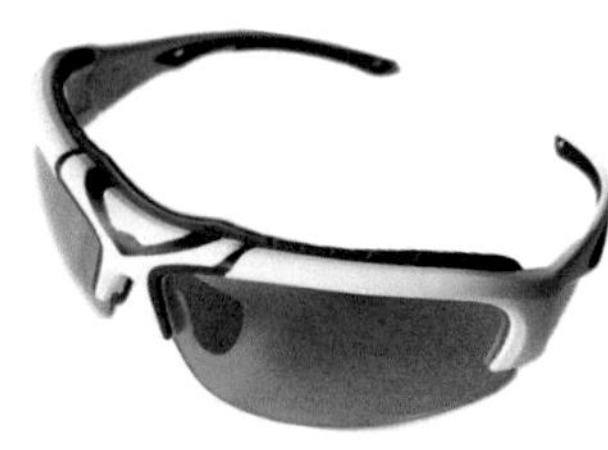

Glasses from LowBlueLights.com block 100% of blue light, $25–$60. Glasses that block 98% of blue light are available from Uvex for as low as $10.

Another way to trick to brain into thinking it's dark out is to use blue light-blocking amber light bulbs (in an otherwise pitch-black room). Smart phones or tablets can be used in an otherwise dark room if set to filter blue light, which is call Night Mode (Android) or Night Shift (iOS), although this setting does not filter as much light as the glasses.

Blue-light-blocking glasses are also useful for insomnia in non-bipolar individuals when worn 1 to 2 hours prior to bedtime. No one should wear the glasses prior to 6 pm because this will mess with circadian rhythms and potentially disrupt mood. Wearing them in the morning could lead to depression. For depression, phototherapy with a light box would be the proper morning time treatment.

There is emerging evidence of a connection between blue light exposure and breast cancer, prostate cancer, obesity, and diabetes.

Henriksen et al. Blue-blocking glasses as additive treatment for mania: a randomized placebo-controlled trial. Bipolar Disord. 2016 May;18[3]:221–32

1912 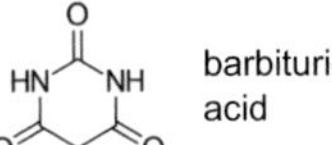 barbituric acid

Barbiturates

bahr BICH er it

"Barb wire"

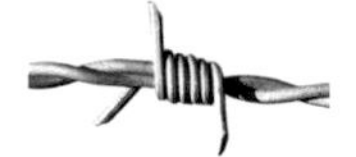

Barbiturates are all derived from barbituric acid, which was discovered on the day of the Feast of Saint Barbara in 1864. Barbiturates, although dangerous, are effective for sleep, anxiety, and seizures. The first medicinal use of a barbiturate was in 1903 when it was discovered barbital would induce sleep in dogs. Shortly thereafter, barbital was marketed as a hypnotic, displacing chloral hydrate for this indication. Barbital is no longer available.

Phenobarbital was discovered in 1911 and hit the market almost immediately as a hypnotic in 1912. In the early 1920s, use of phenobarbital for epilepsy became widespread, eventually displacing potassium bromide for seizure prophylaxis (Yasiry & Shorvon, 2012). Due to safety concerns in the 1960s, benzodiazepines (BZDs/benzos) replaced barbiturates for anxiolytic and hypnotic purposes. However, the average barbiturate is less addictive than the average benzodiazepine because barbiturates have slower onset and longer duration of action.

Compared to BZDs (Chapter 4) barbiturates have a higher risk of death with overdose due to respiratory arrest. While BZDs have an antidote (flumazenil), there is no antidote for a barbiturate overdose. BZDs depress respiration but do not cause death unless combined with alcohol or other sedatives.

Barbiturates are shredders—strong in**D**ucers of CYP450 enzymes. BZDs neither induce nor inhibit. BZDs are only CYP victims, mostly as 3A4 substrates.

Like BZDs, barbiturates bind to GABA(A) receptors at a distinct binding site. While benzodiazepines increase the frequency of chloride channel opening, barbiturates increase the duration of chloride channel opening—think barbiDURate (mnemonic from *Dirty USMLE*). Barbiturates also block glutamate receptors.

All BZDs are regulated as DEA Schedule IV controlled substances. As shown in the table below, some barbiturates are more restricted than others, ranging from Schedule II to non-controlled.

GABA(A) receptor

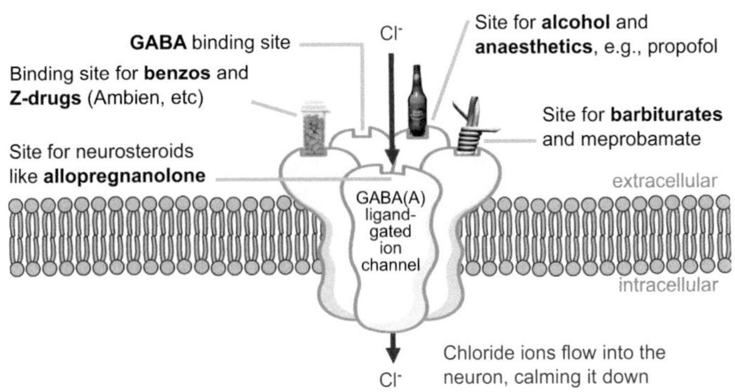

GABA receptor ligands

GABA(A) agonists

- Alcohol
- Ativan, alprazolam, etc (benzos)
- Amytal, etc (barbiturates)
- Ambien, etc (Z-drugs)
- Anesthetics
- Allopregnanolone (brexanolone)

GABA(A) antagonist

- Flumazenil (Romazicon) at the benzodiazepine site

GABA(B) agonists

- Baclofen (antispasmodic)
- GHB (Xyrem)

Note that gabapentin (Neurontin) and pregabalin (Lyrica) have chemical structures similar to GABA but they do **not** bind GABA receptors.

Barbiturate	cost / month	DEA Schedule	Duration of effect	Comments
Phenobarbital (LUMINAL) ← Metabolized to	$40	IV	10–12 hr	Phenobarbital, available since 1912, is the oldest antiepileptic still in use. It is the #10 most prescribed antiepileptic drug. It has a long half-life and can be used to treat withdrawal from alcohol.
Primidone (MYSOLINE)	$15	non-controlled	~ 6 hr	Off-label treatment of tremor; One active metabolite of primidone is phenobarbital.
Butabarbital (BUTISOL)	$140	IV	~ 6 hr	FDA-approved for preoperative sedation and short-term treatment of insomnia; very rarely prescribed
Mephobarbital (MEBARAL)	N/A	II	10–12 hr	Anxiety pill available from 1935, discontinued in 2012
FIORICET butalbital + acetaminophen + caffeine	$20	non-controlled	~ 4 hr	Butalbital is found in combination pills for tension headaches. These combos are not recommended. Butalbital in Fioricet is a common cause of positive drug screens for barbiturates.
FIORICET with codeine	$100	III	~ 4 hr	Will cause positive drug screen for barbiturates (butalbital) and opioids (codeine)
Secobarbital (SECONAL)		II	~ 6 hr	A drug of choice for physician-assisted suicide and the death penalty; The most potent p450 enzyme in**D**ucer of the barbiturate family.
Pentobarbital (NEMBUTAL)		II	~ 6 hr	Used for animal euthanasia and physician-assisted suicide; The pills were known as "yellow jackets".
Amobarbital (AMYTAL)		II	~ 6 hr	Intravenous amobarbital has been called a truth serum. The "Amytal interview" has been used by ER physicians to differentiate between psychiatric and physiologic catatonia-like states.
Thiopental (SODIUM PENTOTHAL)		III	ultra-short 20–30 min	Used for induction of general anesthesia, largely replaced by propofol; Unavailable since 2011, when the European Union banned selling it to countries using it for executions

Phenobarbital (LUMINAL)

1912
$16–$42

fee no BAR bi tal / LUM i nal

"Fear no barbed 'Luminati"

- Barbiturate
- DEA Schedule IV

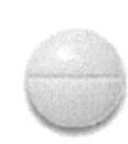

15 mg
16.2
30
32.4
60
64.8
97.2
100

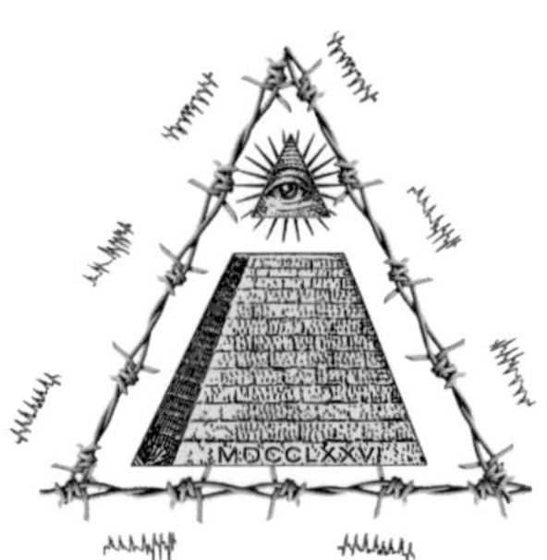

Dosing: For 14-day outpatient benzo detox the initial dose is 30 mg QID, tapered down to 15 mg QID by day 6, then and down to 15 mg QOD by day 10. Do not use for anyone at risk of overdosing.

FDA-approved for:
- Seizure disorder
- Status epilepticus
- Sedation

Used off-label for:
- Alcohol withdrawal
- Benzodiazepine withdrawal

Phenobarbital, brought to market in 1912, was a commonly prescribed sedative and hypnotic until the introduction of benzodiazepines in the 1960s. It is the oldest antiepileptic still in use today. Barbiturates are no longer commonly prescribed for psychiatric purposes. Compared to benzodiazepines, barbiturates have a higher risk of death with overdose due to respiratory arrest. Phenobarbital is less addictive than benzodiazepines because it crosses the blood-brain barrier slowly and is less likely to cause euphoria. It takes over an hour to take effect when taken orally.

Side effects include sedation, cognitive difficulty, and depression. Long term use causes decreased bone mineral density, as is the case with all of the CYP450-inducing "shredder" antiepileptics (phenobarbital, carbamazepine and phenytoin).

Phenobarbital has a long half-life of about 100 hours, allowing once daily dosing. It can be detected in a urine drug screen (UDS) 2–3 weeks after discontinuation. Other barbiturates are only detectable for 2–4 days. Thanks to its long half-life, a phenobarbital taper is useful for management of withdrawal from benzodiazepines (BZDs) or alcohol.

Phenobarbital is one of the active metabolites of primidone, shown below. Phenobarbital is a Schedule IV controlled substance.

Luminal should not be confused with luminol, a chemical used to detect trace amounts of blood at crime scenes. Luminol (not phenobarbital) becomes luminescent upon reaction with the iron in hemoglobin.

Dynamic interactions:
- Sedation/CNS depression

Kinetic interactions:
- Barbiturates are "shredder" inducers of several CYP enzymes, leading to decreased blood levels of countless victim medications.
- 2C19 substrate
- Increased metabolism of thyroid hormone

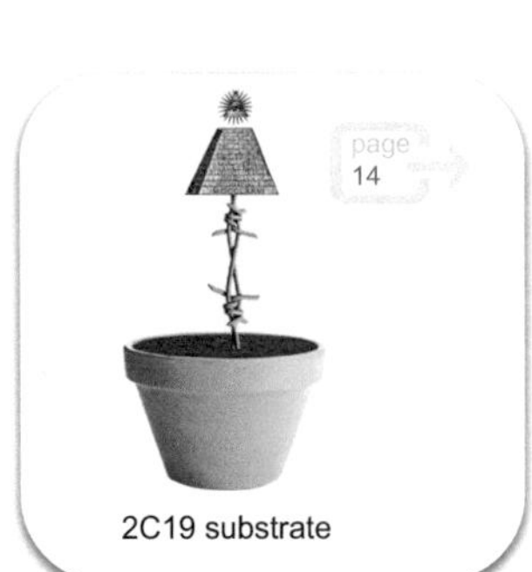

2C19 substrate

page 14

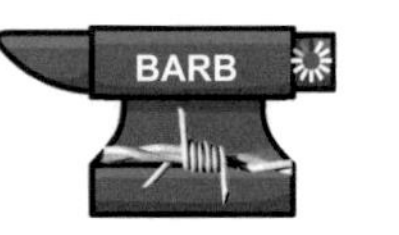

3A4 inducer

page 16

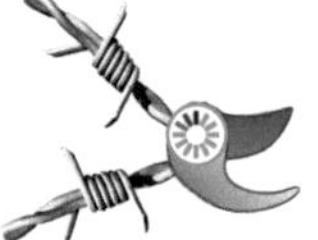

2C19 inducer

page 14

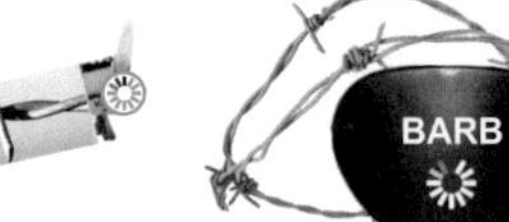

2B6 inducer

page 12

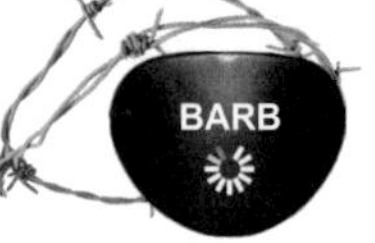

2C9 inducer

page 13

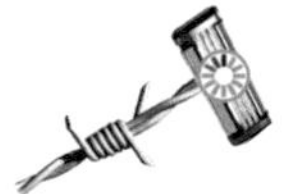

Inducer of lamotrigine metabolism (UGT)

page 17

Primidone (MYSOLINE)

#237
1954
$7–$16

PRIM a dohn / MY soh leen

"Prima donna's Missile line"

- Barbiturate
- Non-controlled

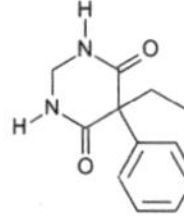

50
250
mg

FDA-approved for:
- Seizure

Used off-label for:
- Essential tremor

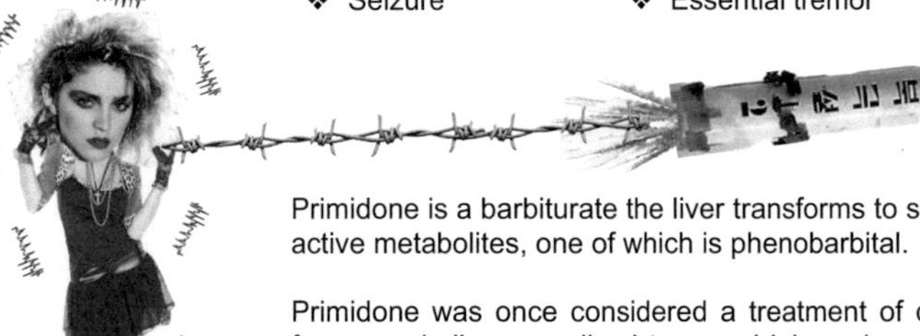

Primidone is a barbiturate the liver transforms to several active metabolites, one of which is phenobarbital.

Primidone was once considered a treatment of choice for secondarily generalized temporal lobe seizures, but it has largely fallen into disuse. It has been withdrawn from various markets around the world but, is still available in the United States. Primidone is a non-controlled substance, despite being metabolized to phenobarbital, which is a Schedule IV controlled substance.

Primidone is effective for essential tremor, but safer options are available today, including benzodiazepines and the beta blocker propranolol (Inderal). Primidone increases clearance of thyroid hormone (T3, T4) and may also have destructive effects on the thyroid gland (Jamshidnezhad & Shariati, 2018). This is an effect likely applicable to phenobarbital also.

Dosing: For essential tremor start 25 mg HS, increase weekly to target dose of 50–250 mg HS; Divide doses > 250 mg/day. Max is 750 mg/day. The target dose for epilepsy is 250 mg TID to QID, with maximum of 2,000 mg/day. Adjust dose based on response and serum levels. As with any antiepileptic, taper gradually when stopping.

The original branded 50 mg tab

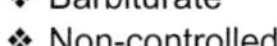

Interactions:
- Same interaction as phenobarbital

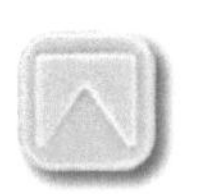

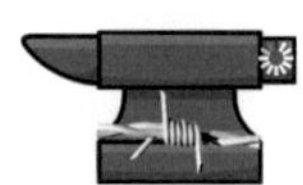

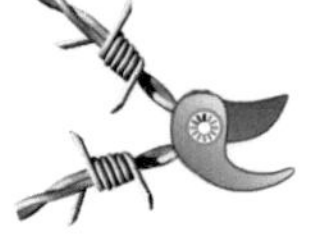

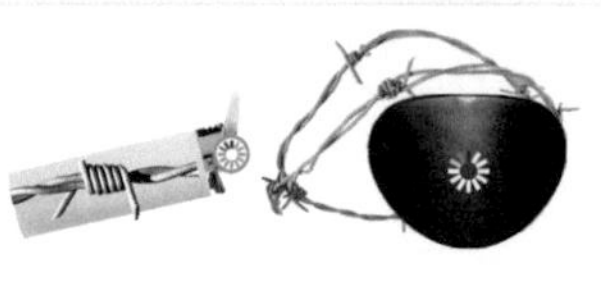

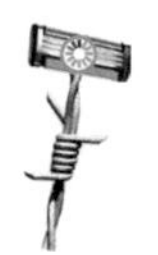

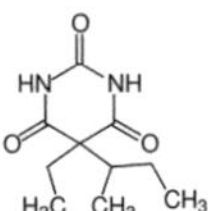

Butabarbital (BUTISOL)

1958
$131–$142

bue ta BAR bi tal / BUE ti sol

"Butter barb"

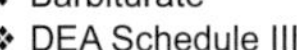

❖ Barbiturate
❖ DEA Schedule III

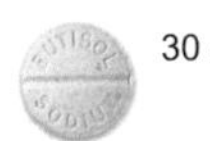

30 mg

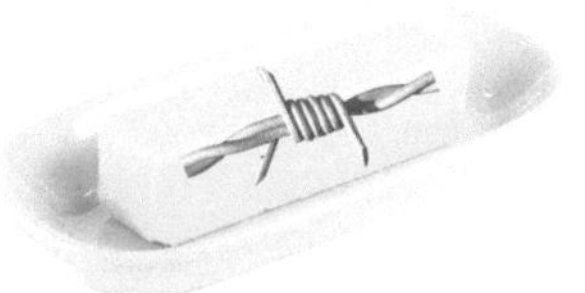

Butabarbital is an intermediate-acting barbiturate FDA-approved for preoperative sedation and short-term treatment of insomnia. It is still available but rarely prescribed. It is a Schedule III controlled substance, which is more restricted than phenobarbital (Schedule IV) but less restricted than the others. In the 1950s and 1960s marketing focused on treatment of female neurosis, although not exclusively—there was a "now he can cope" ad also.

"Mabel is unstable" - 1956

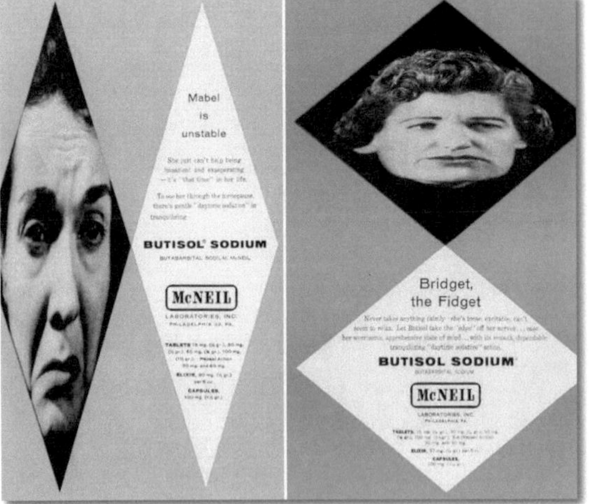

1964

When nervous tension augments family problems

BUTISOL SODIUM
butabarbital sodium

restores composure without loss of responsibility

To help the high-strung, tense patient cope with her problems, BUTISOL SODIUM butabarbital sodium can be used to restore calm without appreciable daytime drowsiness or impairment of mental processes.

In a "clinical re-evaluation" of daytime sedatives, BUTISOL SODIUM butabarbital sodium provided the highest rating (therapeutic index).* Unlike phenobarbital, it does not tend to produce cumulative toxicity.

McNEIL

1969

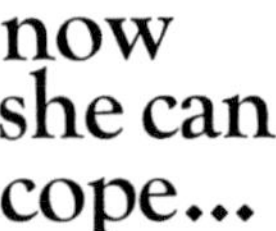

thanks to

Butisol SODIUM
(SODIUM BUTABARBITAL)

"daytime sedative" for everyday situational stress

McNEIL

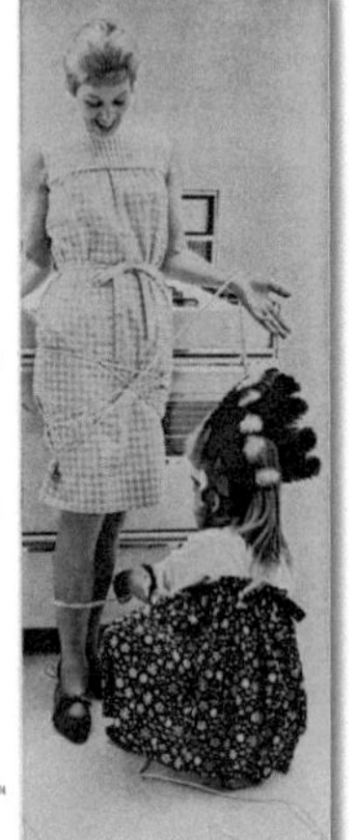

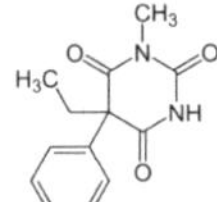

Mephobarbital (MEBARAL)

1935
N/A since 2012

meph o BAR bi tal / MEB a ral

"Mephisto barbed My barrel"

❖ Barbiturate
❖ Off market

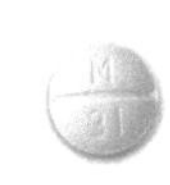

Unavailable

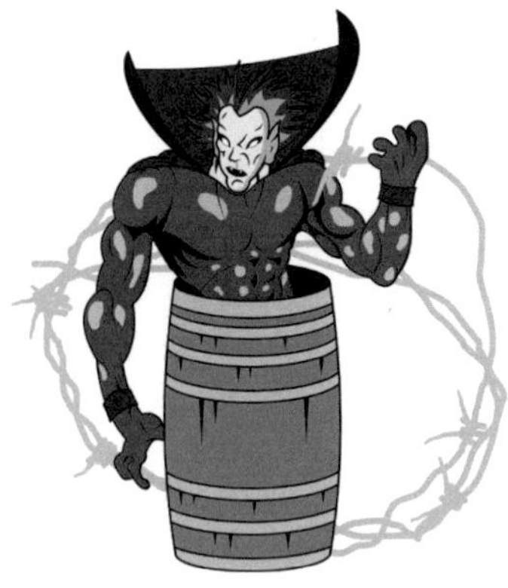

Mephisto is a Marvel comics supervillain

Mephobarbital, also known as methylphenobarbital, was discontinued in 2012 under the Unapproved Drugs Initiative. The FDA was no longer willing to allow the drug to be grandfathered, and the company declined to re-apply for approval. By 2012, its use as an anxiolytic had been mostly abandoned, but a few patients were still taking it as an anticonvulsant.

Decades ago, it was marketed to physicians as a treatment for the patient who "overreacts to any situation". It was a Schedule II controlled substance.

WHEN SHE OVERREACTS TO ANY SITUATION

When the patient tells you that she is too "easily upset," think of Mebaral. Overreaction to everyday occurrences may be a threat to this patient's well-being. Mebaral reduces restlessness and irritability; it has a *familiar* sedative effect. But Mebaral has the advantage of ". . . extremely low incidence of toxicity . . ." and does not produce *sedative daze*. Often physicians prefer the sedative effects of Mebaral to those of phenobarbital.

For daytime sedation – ½ grain, ¾ grain, and occasionally 1½ grains three or four times daily.

MEBARAL

SEDATION WITHOUT SEDATIVE DAZE

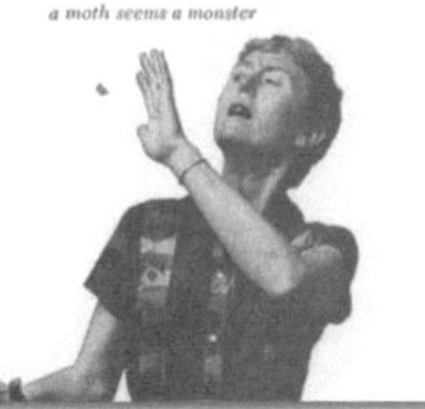

1959

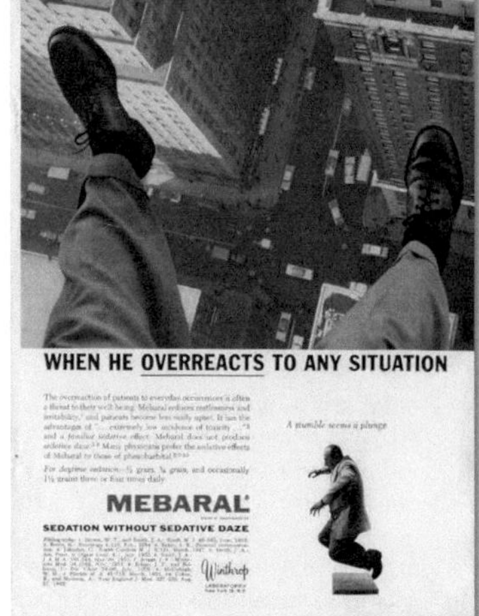

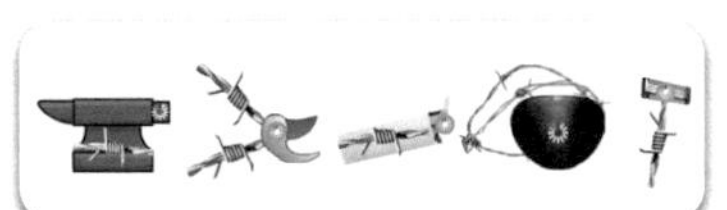

1970
$17–$43

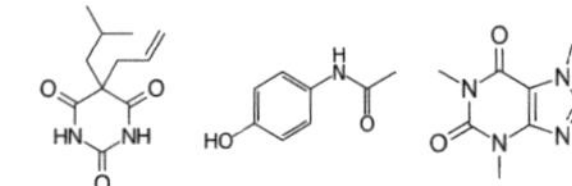

Butalbital combo (FIORICET)

bue TAL bi tal / fee OR a set

"Butane Fire setter"

❖ Headache combo:
- Barbiturate
- Acetaminophen
- Caffeine

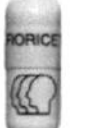

50/325/40 mg

FDA-approved for:
❖ Tension headaches

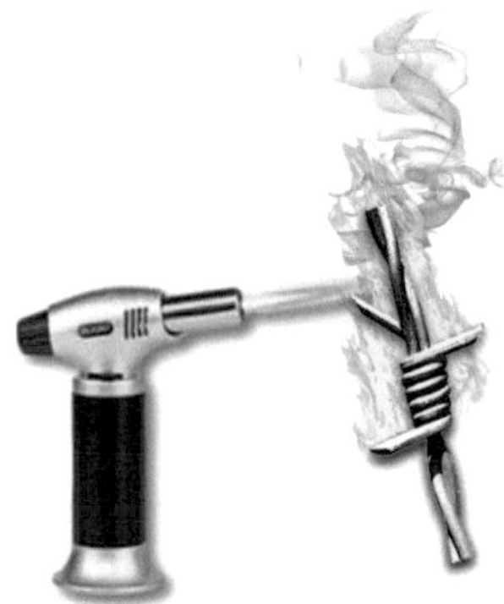

Butalbital is available in combination headache pills, but is not available individually. The butalbital component is included as a sedative. It does not directly help headaches, and may lead to overuse headache. These combos are not recommended. Fioricet is the most common cause of positive drug screens for barbiturates.

The various butalbital combos are FDA-approved for tension headaches, the most common headache type. There is a black box warning, but just regarding risk of hepatotoxicity with > 4,000 mg/day of acetaminophen.

Fioricet = butalbital, acetaminophen, and caffeine—non-controlled substance

Fiorinal = butalbital, aspirin, and caffeine

Fioricet #3 = butalbital, acetaminophen, caffeine, and codeine. It is a Schedule III controlled substance because it contains codeine.

Butalbital is a weaker CYP450 in**D**ucer than phenobarbital.

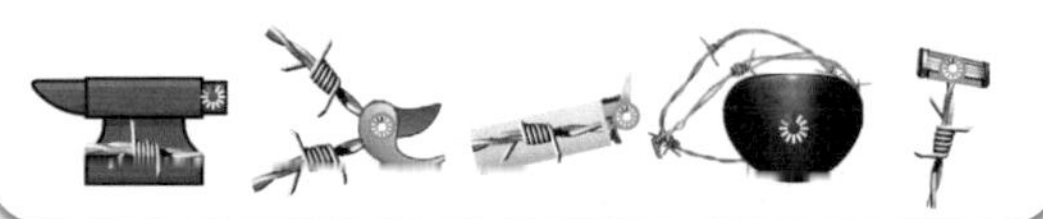

1934
$2,314–$4,317

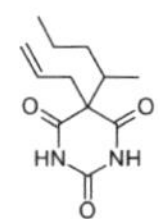

Secobarbital (SECONAL)

SEE ko BAR bi tal / sec on ALL

"Second barb"

❖ Barbiturate
❖ DEA Schedule II

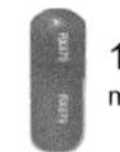

100 mg

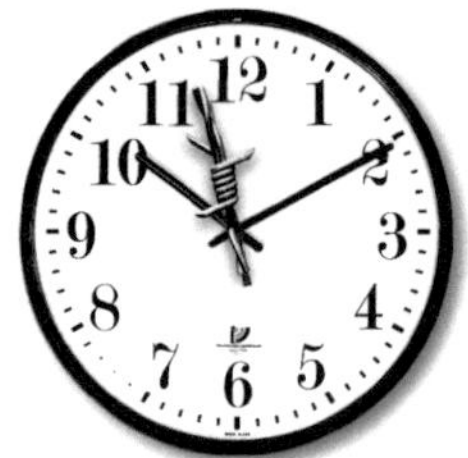

Countdown to death—notice the "barb" is the second hand

Secobarbital is used for physician-assisted suicide. A lethal dose of secobarbital prescribed under Death with Dignity laws recently cost about $4,000.

For death penalty executions, secobarbital (which induces sleep) is given before pancuronium bromide (to paralyze the diaphragm), and potassium chloride (to stop the heart).

The capsules were once widely abused, nicknamed "red devils" or "reds".

Secobarbital is a Schedule II controlled substance, meaning it is more tightly restricted than some other barbiturates.

Among barbiturates, secobarbital is the most potent in**D**ucer of CYP450 enzymes.

Seconal is the most potent CYP inducer of the barbiturates.

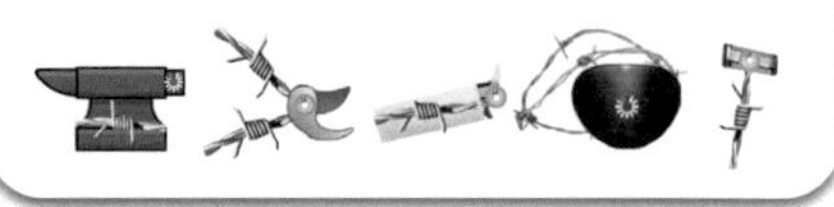

1930
$1,000/gram

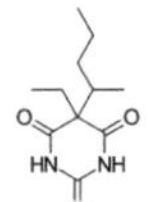

Pentobarbital (NEMBUTAL)

pen toe BAR bi tal / nem bu TAL

"Nimble Pinto"

❖ Barbiturate
❖ DEA Schedule II

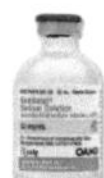

FDA-approved for:
❖ Insomnia (short term use)
—no longer prescribed for sleep
❖ Preoperative sedation

Pentobarbital is a high potency, short acting barbiturate used for physician-assisted suicide, the death penalty, and animal euthanasia (Euthasol brand for dogs). It was originally developed for narcolepsy. Pentobarbital is a Schedule II controlled substance.

Pentobarbital has been used for physician-assisted suicide in California, Colorado, Hawaii, Montana, Oregon, Vermont, and Washington. It has been used for the death penalty in Missouri.

Liquid pentobarbital cost about $500 for a lethal dose (10 grams) until around 2012, when the price rose to about $20,000 due to the European Union's ban on exports to the US for capital punishment. The powder form is still available for only $270 for a lethal dose.

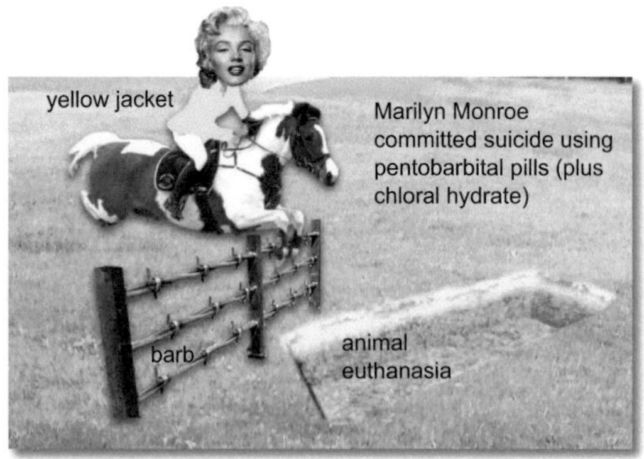

The capsules, no longer available, were widely abused. They were referred to as "yellow jackets".

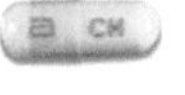

1930
$117 (500 mg vial)

Amobarbital (Amytal)

am oh BAR bi tal / AM a tal

"Am I tall?"

❖ Barbiturate
❖ DEA Schedule II

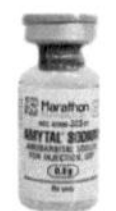

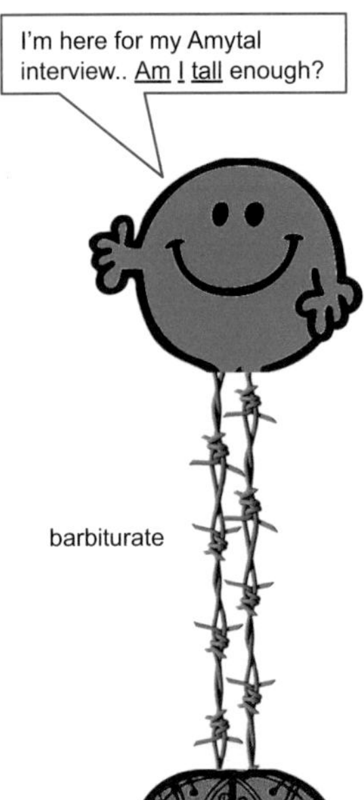

Amobarbital (Amytal) is a Schedule II controlled barbiturate that has been administered intravenously as a "truth serum".

The Amytal interview was introduced in 1930 as a specific technique for administration of IV amobarbital to patients with psychosis. Over the next 20 years, indications for the Amytal Interview multiplied, and the technique became known as "narcosynthesis". The Amytal interview has been used to recover memory in psychogenic amnesia and fugue states, and to treat conversion disorder.

In the emergency department setting, the Amytal interview can be used to evaluate mute, catatonic or stuporous patients in order to differentiate organic from psychogenic causes.

The Amytal interview involves telling the patient the medication is to help him relax and feel like talking. Amobarbital is infused no faster than 50 mg/min to prevent sleep or respiratory depression. The infusion continues until either rapid lateral nystagmus is present or drowsiness is noted, which usually requires 150–130 mg. The infusion continues at 5–10 mg/min until the interview is concluded (Perry & Jacobs, 1982). The expected total amount of amobarbital needed is in the ballpark of 500–750 mg.

For surgical patients about to undergo a temporal lobectomy (for refractory epilepsy), amobarbital is used to determine which side of the brain controls language and memory. This technique is called the intracarotid sodium amobarbital procedure (ISAP) or Wada test (WAH-duh), named for the surgeon who invented it. The procedure is done by injecting amobarbital into the right or left internal carotid artery to put that hemisphere of the brain to sleep. If the epileptic focus is in the dominant hemisphere, the patient is a poor surgical candidate.

The pills, nicknamed Blue 88s were given to battle fatigued US soldiers in World War II. It allowed the soldier to relax for a couple of days before returning to front-line duties. The capsules are no longer available.

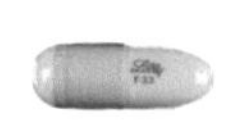

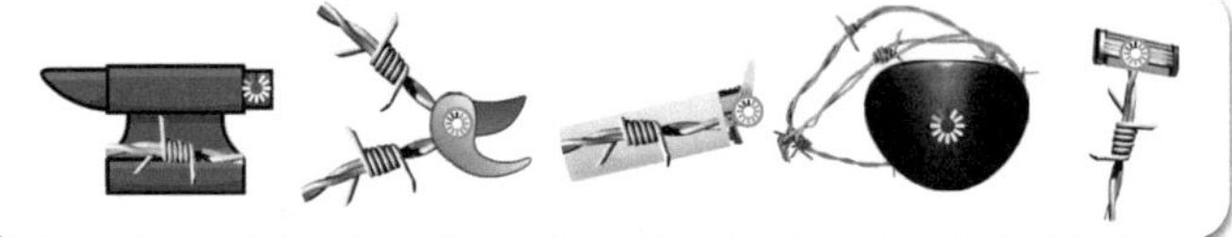

1934
Unavailable since 2011

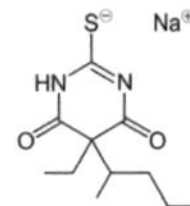

Thiopental (Sodium Pentothal)

thi oh PENT al / PENT o thal

"Tire Penthouse"

❖ Barbiturate
❖ DEA Schedule III

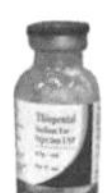

Unavailable

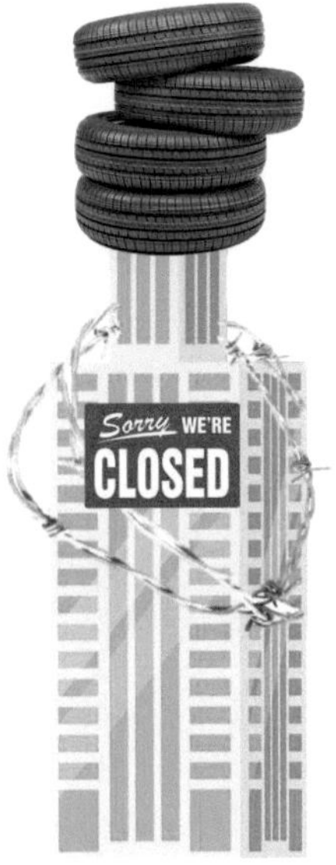

Sodium thiopental is ultra-short-acting barbiturate and a Schedule III controlled substance. It was used in the induction phase of general anesthesia, although it has been largely replaced by propofol. With an IV infusion, consciousness is lost in 30 to 45 seconds and returns in 5 to 10 minutes.

Thiopental is used intravenously for physician-assisted suicide to induce coma. It is typically followed by pancuronium bromide which paralyzes the diaphragm thus stopping respiration. In 2009 Ohio became the first state to use a one-drug method for the death penalty, that drug being thiopental.

In 2011 sodium thiopental was removed from the US market due to a European Union ban. The ban was in response to America's use of the drug for death penalty executions. This prompted the American Society of Anesthesiologists to release a statement about being "extremely troubled", characterizing the ban on this "critical drug" as an important patient safety issue. Until 2011, sodium thiopental was still considered a first-line anesthetic in many cases.

Thiopental is a Schedule III controlled substance.

Dynamic interactions:
❖ Sedation/CNS depression

Kinetic interactions:
❖ Barbiturates are "shredder" inducers of several CYP enzymes, leading to decreased blood levels of countless victim medications.
❖ Increased metabolism of thyroid hormone

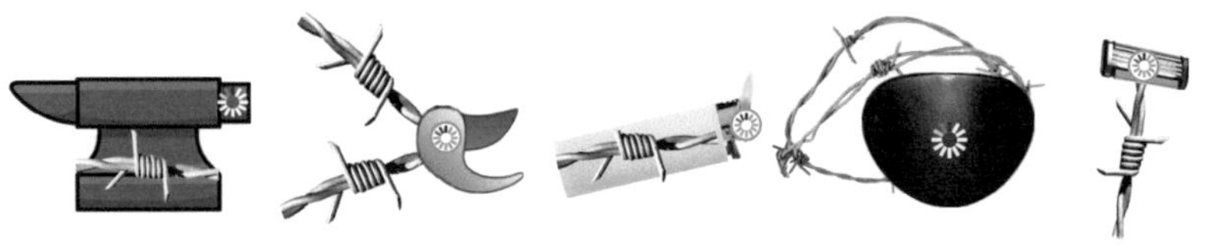

Visit cafermed.com and use promo code **EMBIGGEN** for a discount on the big book, Cafer's Psychopharmacology: Visualize to Memorize 270 Medication Mascots.

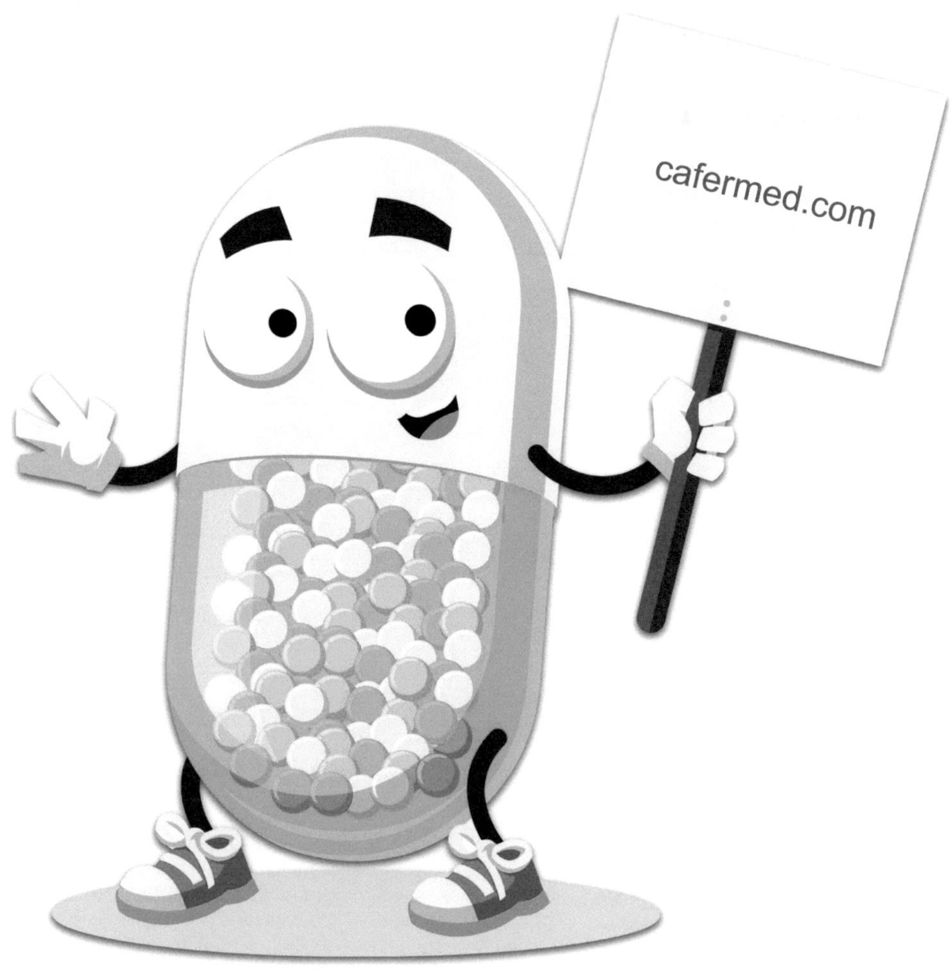

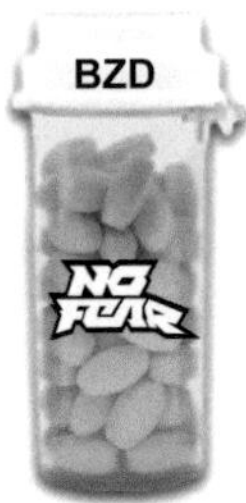

Never "been so" calm. Benzodiazepines (BZDs/benzos) comprise the main class of sedatives used for short-term relief of generalized anxiety disorder (GAD), panic disorder, and social anxiety disorder. About 10% of adults have taken a benzodiazepine over the course of a year. They are the second-most abused class of prescription drugs, behind opioids. The core structure of a BZD is a benzene ring fused to a seven-membered diazepine ring. Members of the BZD class are similar, varying in duration of action, speed of onset, and tendency to accumulate in the body.

BZDs are indirect GABA(A) receptor agonists that alter the configuration of the receptor, increasing the receptor's affinity for GABA. GABA is the main neurotransmitter involved in inhibiting neuronal activity in the brain.

GABA(A) receptor

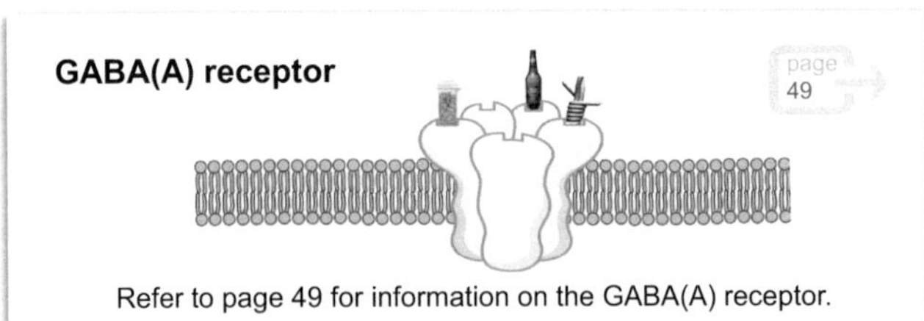

Refer to page 49 for information on the GABA(A) receptor.

All BZDs are Schedule IV controlled substances (less strictly restricted than opioids or ADHD stimulants, which are Schedule II). Due to their addictive nature, BZDs are intended for short-term use. If used for long-term treatment, BZDs are ideally taken PRN on non-consecutive days. Otherwise, efficacy is diminished as tolerance develops. For long term treatment of anxiety, SSRI or SNRI antidepressants are preferable. Stopping (or even decreasing the dose of) a chronically used BZD is difficult due to withdrawal symptoms and rebound anxiety. Individuals continuing a BZD for 3 years were more anxious and depressed than those whose BZD was stopped (Rickels et al, 1991). BZDs are ineffective and potentially harmful for the treatment of PTSD and phobias. BZD treatment increases the incidence of psychiatric hospitalization.

The main side effects of BZDs are sedation, fatigue, and forgetfulness. There are few side effects otherwise. BZDs do not affect metabolic parameters (weight, glucose tolerance, etc), are not anticholinergic, and do not require laboratory monitoring. Benzodiazepines are significantly safer than barbiturates, which were the predominant anxiolytics prior to the 1960s. BZD overdose is usually not fatal. However, they can lead to respiratory arrest in combination with alcohol and opioids. BZDs should not be co-prescribed with opioids. They are particularly dangerous in combination with methadone.

BZDs should be used only with extreme caution by patients with sleep apnea. From 2006–2008 BZDs were not covered by Medicare Part D due to risk of hip fracture from falls. BZDs can cause behavioral disinhibition, similar to how alcohol can lead to bar fights. Rarely, BZDs have caused acute rage reactions.

Benzos are akin to "alcohol in pill" in that ethanol also binds to the GABA(A) receptor, although at a different distinct site. BZD and alcohol dependence is a result of a conformational change to the GABA(A) receptor that decreases its affinity for GABA. Medically, alcohol withdrawal and BZD withdrawal are essentially the same condition. Withdrawal symptoms can include tremor, sweating, nausea/vomiting, and perceptual disturbances (tactile, auditor, and/or visual). Management of either type of withdrawal includes substituting a long-acting BZD or barbiturate dosed according to symptoms.

Withdrawal symptoms from stopping a BZD can occur after 4 weeks of continuous use. BZD withdrawal onset is within 12–48 hours, depending on the half-life of the BZD being stopped. Intensity of withdraw peaks in intensity around days 1–5. Duration of withdrawal can extend 7–21 days.

A black box warning advises concomitant use of BZDs and opioids triples the risk of opioid-related fatalities. Long-term BZD use is associated with a 2-fold increase in development of dementia, although the absence of a dose-response association argues against causality (Gray et al, 2016).

For patients established on high dose BZD treatment, discontinuation should be by slow taper over 4 to 8 weeks. Since BZDs are antiepileptics, abrupt discontinuation can precipitate a seizure. Withdrawal from BZDs, barbiturates, or alcohol can be fatal. This is not the case with withdrawal from other classes of addictive drugs.

BZDs are necessary for treatment of alcohol-withdrawal delirium (in combination with an antipsychotic). BZDs may worsen other types of delirium. Delirium from any etiology can be managed with an antipsychotic with minimal anticholinergic properties such as haloperidol, aripiprazole, quetiapine, risperidone, or ziprasidone.

BZDs are useful for acute mania, in combination with a mood stabilizer and an antipsychotic. Some experts regard BZDs as the first-line option for treatment of tardive dyskinesia. BZDs are the first-line treatment for catatonia, a stuporous condition with odd mannerisms and little response to external stimuli. The "lorazepam challenge" test (page 58) can help elucidate whether catatonia is due to psychological or organic factors.

There are three available BZDs that do not need to be metabolized by CYP enzymes—Lorazepam, Oxazepam and Temazepam = "**LOT**". These three BZDs are preferable for the elderly and those with hepatic insufficiency.

Metabolism of the non-LOT BZDs is through oxidation, catalyzed by CYP enzymes. Since the liver's ability to oxidize (Phase I metabolism) declines with age, the elderly are especially sensitive to the accumulation of non-LOT BZDs.

The three "LOT" BZDs are metabolized by conjugation with glucuronide (Phase II metabolism). The liver's Phase II metabolic capability does not significantly decline with age. LOT benzos are substrates of UGT2B15, which is inhibited of valproate (Depakote). Valproate can double blood levels of lorazepam.

BZDs are 3A4 substrates

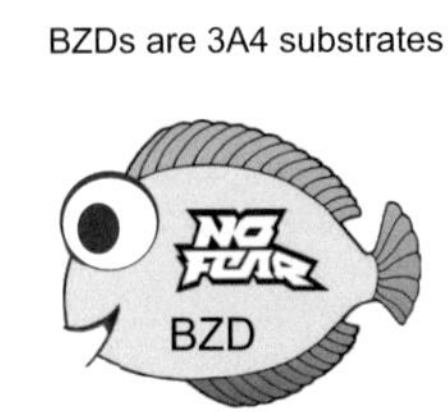

Excluding:

- **L**orazepam (Ativan)
- **O**xazepam (Serax)
- **T**emazepam (Restoril)
- Clobazam (Onfi) - 2C19

These **3A4 inDucers** can reduce blood levels of most BZDs:

- Carbamazepine (Tegretol)
- Efavirenz (Sustiva)
- Modafinil (Provigil)
- Nevirapine (Viramune)
- Oxcarbazepine (Trileptal)
- Phenobarbital (Luminal)
- Phenytoin (Dilantin)
- Rifampin (Rifadin)
- St John's Wort

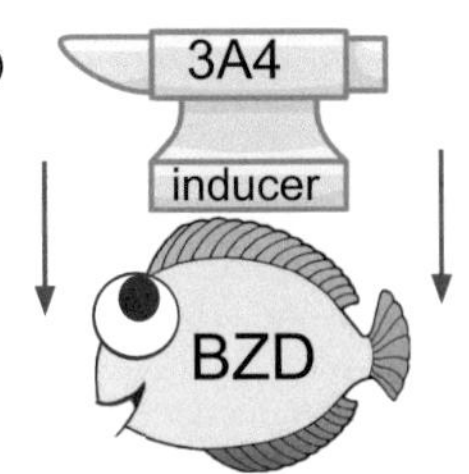

3A4 inHibitors increase blood levels of most BZDs, potentially resulting in oversedation.

- Grapefruit juice
- Protease Inhibitors (HIV)
- Cimetidine (Tagamet)
- Clarithromycin (Biaxin)
- Diltiazem (Cardizem)
- Erythromycin
- Fluconazole (Diflucan)
- Fluoxetine (Prozac)
- Fluvoxamine (Luvox)
- Itraconazole (Sporanox)
- Ketoconazole (Nizoral)
- Nefazodone (Serzone)

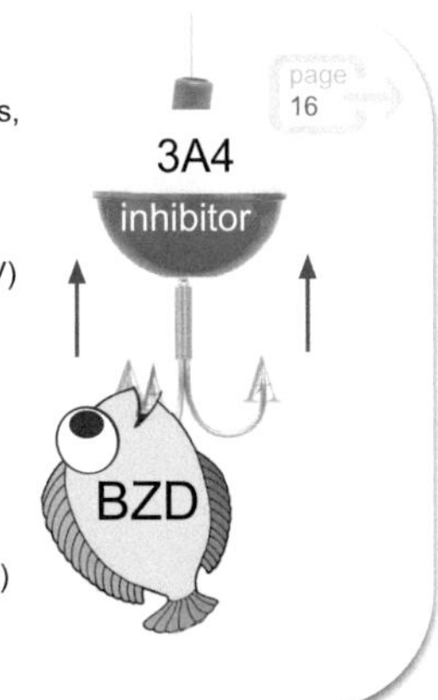

Benzodiazepines used for anxiety (anxiolytics) and/or insomnia (hypnotics)

#Rx	Benzodiazepine (approx cost/month)	Onset*	Duration	mg equiv	Details
#1	Alprazolam (XANAX) $10 Xanax XR $15 Alprazolam ODT $10	rapid	short	0.5	The most prescribed, least sedating, and most addictive BZD; High risk of seizures if suddenly discontinued due to short half-life XR = extended-release; ODT = orally disintegrating table
#2	Clonazepam (KLONOPIN) $10	med	med/long	0.25–0.5	Similar effect to lorazepam but with longer half-life and vulnerability to CYP interactions as a 3A4 substrate
#3	Lorazepam (ATIVAN) $10 Lorazepam IM (per dose) $10	med	short/med	1	The first-line BZD for anxiety, especially in the elderly and individuals with liver disease; No CYP interactions
#4	Diazepam (VALIUM) $10	rapid	long	5	Addictive due to rapid onset; used for alcohol withdrawal due to long half-life
#5	Temazepam (RESTORIL) $10	slow	med	15	The original branded capsules have "for sleep" printed on them.
#6	Chlordiazepoxide (LIBRIUM) $15	med	long	25	The first benzo (1960); useful for alcohol withdrawal due to long half-life
#7	Triazolam (HALCION) $50	med	short	0.25–0.5	#1 prescribed sleep medication until 1990s when shown to be more dangerous than other BZDs
#8	Clorazepate (TRANXENE) $100	med	long	7.5	Marketed as an anxiolytic with less sedation
#9	Oxazepam (SERAX) $100	slow	short	15	Lowest potential for abuse and lowest fatality index due to slow onset
#10	Flurazepam (DALMANE) $25	med	long	15	For insomnia but half-life is too long, tends to accumulate
#11	Estazolam (PROSOM) $50	med	med	1	For insomnia, rarely prescribed
#12	Quazepam (DORAL) $500	med	long	7.5	For insomnia, rarely prescribed

*Rapid onset—within 15 minutes. Slow onset 30–60 minutes. Duration of action is generally shorter than plasma half-life. Note that onset of action can be expedited by taking the BZD sublinguilly, which allows directly entry into blood, bypassing first-pass metabolism through the liver.

Other benzodiazepines

Benzo	Onset	Half-life	Details
Clobazam (ONFI) $750	rapid	long	Approved in 2011 for seizures due to Lennox-Gastaut syndrome; used for anxiety in other countries; It is the only available BZD with a 1,5 diazepine ring (rather than 1,4).
Midazolam (VERSED) $15	rapid	short	IV route for general anesthesia and sedation while on mechanical ventilation; the only water-soluble BZD, making it suitable for intranasal treatment of seizures; not available PO
Flunitrazepam (ROHYPNOL)	rapid	long	Similar to diazepam; infamous "Roofie" date rape drug; not sold in the US but available for prescription in Mexico for anxiety and insomnia. Travelers to the US can bring a 30-day supply if declared to customs.

Other GABA(A) ligands (not benzos)

Flumazenil	The antidote for BZD overdose; GABA(A) receptor antagonist at the BZD binding site
Barbiturates	Phenobarbital, primidone, butalbital and other "-barbitals"; In addition to binding GABA(A) receptors, barbiturates block glutamate receptors
Chloral hydrate (NOCTEC)	Discovered in the 1830s, this was the first true hypnotic drug. Chloral hydrate was a popular sleep medication until superseded by the barbiturates in the early 1900s. It is dangerous due to respiratory depression. Chloral hydrate has been unavailable since 2013 when the manufacturer voluntarily withdrew it from market. Prior to 2013 it was available in liquid-filled capsules as a Schedule IV controlled substance, although it was not FDA-approved for any indication. An alcoholic beverage laced with chloral hydrate was known as a "Mickey Finn". To "slip a Mickey" is to give someone these "knockout drops" without their knowledge to incapacitate them. Mr. Finn was a bartender accused of slipping Mickeys to rob customers, circa 1903. Chloral hydrate does not disrupt sleep architecture and does not cause withdrawal.
Methaqualone (Quāālud)	A multifaceted GABA(A) receptor modulator, Quāālude [KWAY - lude] was a popular prescription sedative in the 1970s. Its trade name derived from "quiet interlude" and stylized after Maalox, a widely-used antacid from the same manufacturer. It was discontinued in 1984 after becoming infamous for addictiveness and recreational abuse. Bill Cosby allegedly put 'ludes in womens' drinks for date-rape purposes.
Propofol (DIPRIVAN)	Milky white IV anesthetic, nicknamed "milk of amnesia". Michael Jackson's personal physician administered propofol to Jackson on a regular basis for sleep. Authorities believe the doctor fell asleep while the drug was being administered and may have awakened to find Jackson dead.
Meprobamate (MILTOWN)	Released in 1955, meprobamate was the first blockbuster psychotropic drug. It was referred to as a "minor tranquilizer" (anxiolytic) to distinguish it from the major tranquilizers (antipsychotics). Meprobamate is rarely prescribed today. The muscle relaxant carisoprodol (Soma).

GABA(B) ligands

Baclofen (LIORESAL)	Baclofen is a muscle relaxant that activates GABA(B) receptors *("B" for baclofen)*, relieving spasticity without producing euphoria or pleasant effects. Baclofen is associated with a withdrawal syndrome similar to benzodiazepines or alcohol. It is an effective off-label maintenance treatment of alcohol use disorder.
Xyrem (GHB; sodium oxybate)	Sodium salt of the club drug gamma-hydroxybutyric acid (GHB), approved for narcolepsy/cataplexy. It is an agonist at GHB receptors and GABA(B) receptors. GHB is present in the body naturally in small amounts, and can be obtained illegally for recreational and date rape purposes.

#19
1981
$9–$36
$17–$70 ER

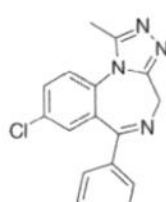

Alprazolam (XANAX)

al PRAY zuh LAM / ZAN ax

"Lil Xan, the Alp-raised Lamb"

- ❖ Benzodiazepine
- ❖ Rapid onset
- ❖ Short duration
- ❖ DEA Schedule IV

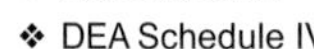
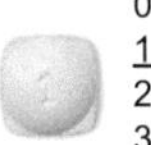

0.5 ER
1 ER
2 ER
3 ER
mg

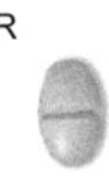
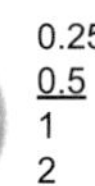

0.25
0.5
1
2
mg

FDA-approved for:

- ❖ Anxiety 0.5 mg TID–1 mg QID
- ❖ Panic disorder 0.5 mg TID–3 mg TID

Used off-label for:

- ❖ Insomnia

The stage name of Lil Xan, a rapper with face tattoos rising to fame in 2017, originated from his addiction to this benzo.

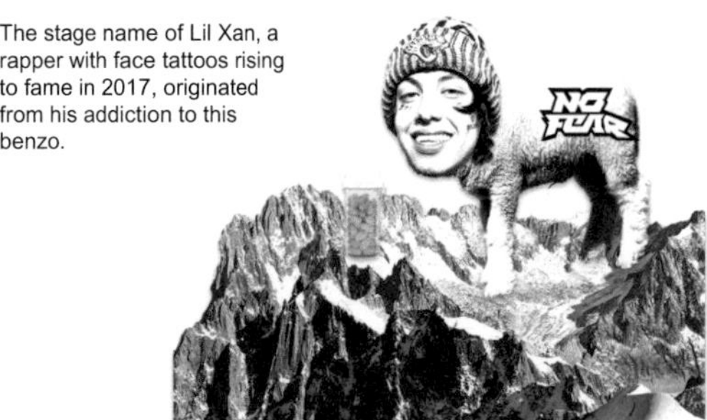

The 2 mg Xanax "bar" is the strongest anxiety pill available. On the street a 2 mg bar is referred to as a "Xanny bar" or, if yellow, a "school bus", sold for about $4 each.

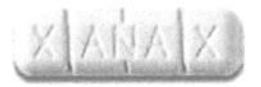

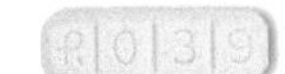

Released in 1981 for panic disorder, alprazolam remains the most prescribed benzodiazepine (BZD), particularly among primary care physicians. Psychiatrists are more likely to choose less addictive BZDs such as clonazepam (Klonopin) or lorazepam (Ativan). Xanax has the advantage of causing the least sedation among BZDs. It can be effective for panic attacks unresponsive to other BZDs. To spell the trade name correctly, think *"X for anXiety".*

Xanax should not be used first-line because it is more habit forming than other benzos. It relieves anxiety "too well", which reinforces dependence on a quick fix and potentially interferes with development of healthy coping skills. Prescribed in small quantity, Xanax is a suitable PRN for infrequent panic attacks or specific phobias such as fear of flying.

Xanax fits the profile of an addictive substance, i.e., quick onset and short duration of action short—the same reasons intravenous drugs and cigarettes are so addictive. The rapid rise of alprazolam levels in the CNS can induce euphoric feelings. Although the elimination half-life of alprazolam is 12 hours, the duration of action is much shorter, requiring TID dosing if taken on a scheduled basis. Xanax's short duration of action may lead to patients "watching the clock" in anticipation of the next available dose.

For context: Presuming oral route of administration, Xanax tends to be more addictive than PO amphetamine (Adderall) but less addictive than opioids (hydrocodone, oxycodone, etc).

It is not recommended to prescribe Xanax to individuals with a significant history of abusing alcohol or recreational drugs. Patients who doctor shop for Xanax are also likely to seek opioids. Benzodiazepines in general increase the risk of opioid-related fatalities 3-fold. Such patients may request Xanax bars by name, often persistently, claiming nothing else works. They may claim to be "allergic" to other weaker benzos and non-addictive anxiolytics such as hydroxyzine (Vistaril) and buspirone (Buspar). A clinic in Louisville KY stopped writing scripts for Xanax altogether because doctors tired of "funneling a great deal of your energy into pacifying, educating, bumping heads with people over Xanax". *"All of my patients ask for alprazolam"* —Madalyn Hoke, PA-S

Although Xanax reduces seizure risk when taken regularly, it should not be prescribed to patients with seizure disorder. Overall, Xanax is associated with a higher risk of seizures than most psychotropic medications. Seizures occur during the withdrawal phase, owing to Xanax's short half-life. Xanax XR is less likely to cause withdrawal seizures.

An individual established on ≥ 4 mg/day of alprazolam is likely physically and psychologically dependent on the medication, and an interruption in supply may be catastrophic from rebound anxiety.

The extended-release (ER) formulation, Xanax XR, is less addictive because the onset is slower, and the therapeutic effect wears off more gradually. Xanax XR is a long-acting BZD, with a duration of action longer than clonazepam (Klonopin). For a patient needing scheduled daily Xanax, the XR formulation may be the way to go.

Alprazolam appears to have antidepressant properties, which cannot be said about other benzos.

Due to short half-life, Xanax may be undetectable by a urine drug screen at 24 hours. Contrast this with long-acting BZDs like chlordiazepoxide (Librium) and diazepam (Valium), which can potentially be detected at one week.

Dosing: Approved range for panic disorder is 0.5–3 mg TID, which allows a very high max of 9 mg/day. The max for anxiety disorder (without panic) is 4 mg/day. You may divide dose to QID if interdose symptoms occur with TID dosing. Taper dose by no more than 0.5 mg/day q 3 days to discontinue. Doing the math, a patient on the maximum of 9 mg/day needs to be tapered off over 2 months. Consider treating alprazolam discontinuation like an alcohol detox using chlordiazepoxide (Librium). With Xanax XR, start at 1 mg QD for max of 6 mg QD.

Dynamic interactions applicable to all benzodiazepines:

- ❖ Sedation/CNS depression
  - Black box warning combing benzodiazepine and opioids may result in respiratory depression, coma, and death
  - Do not combine with alcohol

page 16

Kinetic interactions:

- ❖ 3A4 substrate (major)
  - Alprazolam levels may be doubled by fluvoxamine (Luvox), which a strong 3A4 inHibitor
  - Alprazolam levels are modestly elevated by grapefruit juice (weak 3A4 inHibitor)
  - Alprazolam levels are significantly decreased by potent 3A4 inDucers such as carbamazepine (Tegretol)

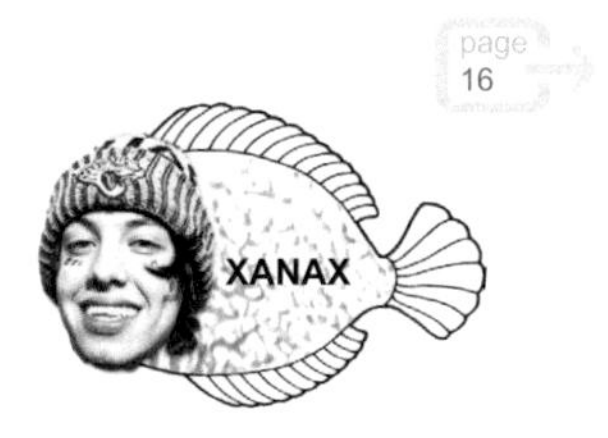

3A4 substrate (major)

#42
1975
$9–$38

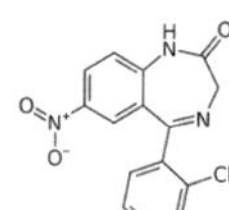

Clonazepam (KLONOPIN)

kloh NEY zuh pam / KLON o pin

"Cloned pin"

- ❖ Benzodiazepine
- ❖ Intermediate onset
- ❖ Intermediate/Long duration
- ❖ DEA Schedule IV

0.5
1
2
mg

FDA approved for:

- ❖ Seizure disorder
- ❖ Panic disorder

Used off-label for:

- ❖ Generalized anxiety disorder
- ❖ Anxious distress of depression
- ❖ Mania (adjunct)
- ❖ Akathisia
- ❖ Insomnia
- ❖ Tardive dyskinesia
- ❖ Catatonia
- ❖ Restless legs syndrome
- ❖ Night terrors
- ❖ REM sleep behavior disorder
- ❖ Tourette's disorder

Clonazepam (Klonopin) is less addictive than alprazolam (Xanax) because its onset is less rapid, and the effect wears off more gradually. Clonazepam is less sedating than the average benzo.

Clonazepam may have anti-manic properties distinct from sedation, making it useful as an adjunct for bipolar mania. For the hospitalized manic patient, a useful trio is clonazepam, plus an antipsychotic and a mood stabilizer. Ideally, clonazepam is tapered off prior to discharge from the hospital.

For benzodiazepines in general, duration of effect is much shorter than half-life. For clonazepam, half-life is 30–40 hours but duration of action is only 6–12. Clonazepam can be detected in blood for over 6 days (half-life x5). Nonetheless, standard drug screens may produce false negative results with clonazepam.

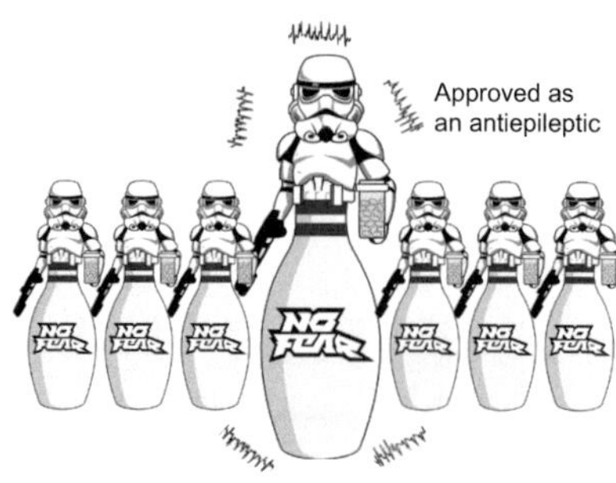

Klonopin wafers are a special formulation designed for sublingual administration. They take effect in 10–20 minutes. Standard PO clonazepam kicks in within 30– 60 minutes when swallowed.

Dosing: For anxiety disorders, start 0.25 mg BID, increase by 0.25 mg/day every 1–2 days for FDA max of 4 mg/day. It is best not to exceed 2 mg/day. Consider PRN dosing, e.g. 4x/week. For acute mania (adjunct) start at least 0.5 mg BID and increase by 0.5 mg/day every 1–2 days, taper prior to discharge. As for any anticonvulsant, taper to discontinue.

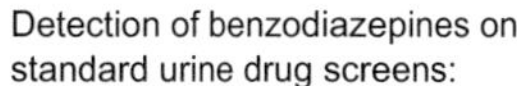

Detection of benzodiazepines on standard urine drug screens:

Usually detected:
Diazepam (Valium)
Alprazolam (Xanax)
- although short half-life

Sometimes missed:
Lorazepam (Ativan)

Commonly missed:
Clonazepam (Klonopin)

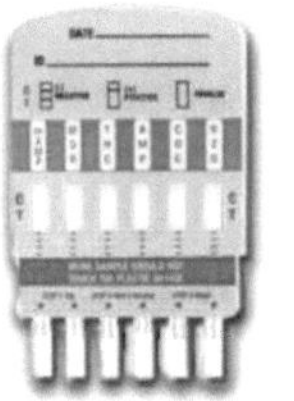

The original branded 1 mg tab

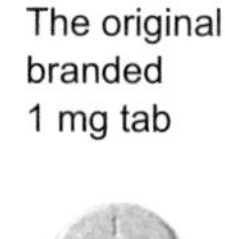

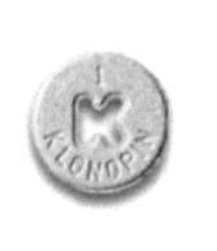

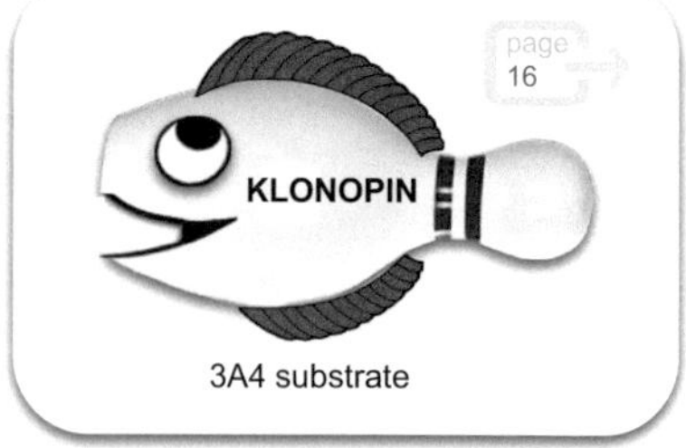

page 16

3A4 substrate

#57
1977
$9–$44

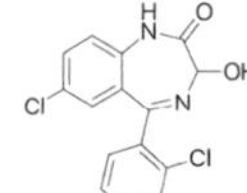

Lorazepam (ATIVAN)

lor az e pam / AT uh van

"Lorax's ATV"

- ❖ Benzodiazepine
- ❖ Intermediate onset
- ❖ Intermediate/Short duration
- ❖ DEA Schedule IV

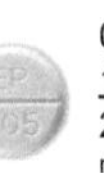

0.5
1
2
mg

FDA-approved for:

- ❖ Anxiety
- ❖ Insomnia (short term treatment)
- ❖ Status epilepticus (IM, IV)

Used off-label for:

- ❖ Same as with clonazepam

If a benzo is necessary, lorazepam is a good choice. Lorazepam does not have an overly long half-life and there are no active metabolites to accumulate.

Ativan is a BZD of choice for those with liver disease and older adults because it metabolized by phase II conjugation only (as opposed by being oxidized by CYP enzymes).

Lorazepam is the only BZD commonly used for IM injection. For intravenous infusion, three benzos are available: lorazepam, diazepam (Valium), and midazolam (Versed).

For acute agitation in an aggressive patient, Ativan 2 mg IM can be coadministered with haloperidol (Haldol) 5 mg IM, a combo health care professionals refer to as a "five and two".

In treatment of epilepsy, lorazepam can be prescribed as a rescue medication for patients who have clusters of seizures It works reasonably quickly when taken orally and the anti-seizure effect lasts for 2 to 6 hours. A lorazepam concentrate of 2 mg (1 ml of liquid) can be taken sublingually in urgent situations (Dr. Robert Fisher, epilepsy.com).

Benzodiazepines are the mainstay of treatment for catatonia, a stuporous condition with odd mannerisms and little response to external stimuli. The "lorazepam challenge" test can help elucidate whether catatonia is due to psychological or organic factors. Upon intravenous administration of 1–2 mg of lorazepam, there may be a marked improvement of catatonia within 10 minutes. A mute patient may be able to speak. A positive lorazepam challenge confirms the diagnosis of catatonia of psychiatric etiology (McEvoy JP, 1986).

Dosing: For anxiety, start 1 mg PO BID or TID. FDA max is 10 mg/day, try not to exceed 4–6 mg/day. For insomnia, start 2 mg ½ to 1 tab HS PRN. For acute mania, start 2 mg TID and taper off as mania improves; For status epilepticus, give 4 mg IV or IM x 1. The standard IM dose for acute agitation is 2 mg. It may be coadministered with Haldol 5 mg IM.

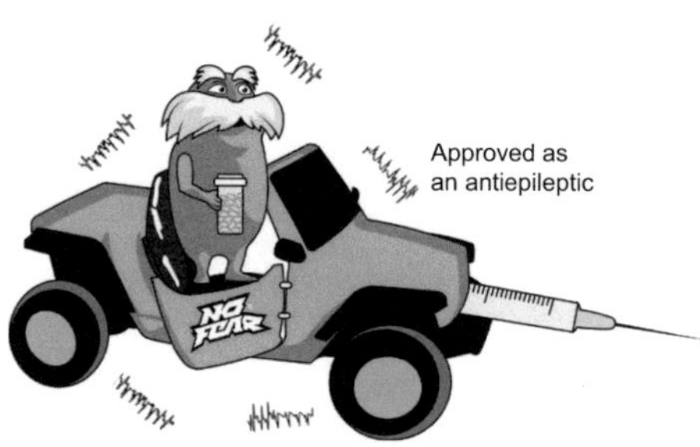

Ativan is the only BZD commonly available for IM injection. It is the preferred IM to abort a seizure.

Dynamic interactions:

- ❖ Sedation
- ❖ Respiratory depression
- ❖ Do not combine with alcohol or opioids

Kinetic interactions:

- ❖ UGT2B15 substrate
  - Lorazepam blood levels can be doubled by valproate (Depakote)

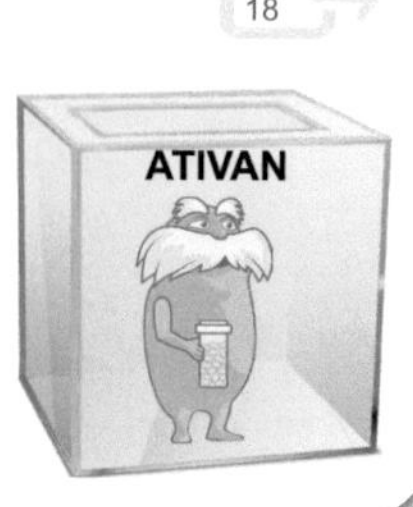

page 18

#112
1963
$6–$12

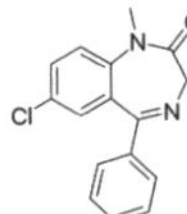

Diazepam (VALIUM)

die AZ uh pam / VAL ee um

"Daisy & Pam (are) Valley (girls)"

- Benzodiazepine
- Rapid onset
- Long duration
- DEA Schedule IV

2
5
10
mg

FDA-approved for:

- Anxiety (PO)
- Preoperative sedation (IM)
- Sedation for cardioversion (IV)
- Sedation for endoscopy (IV)
- Alcohol withdrawal (PO, IV)
- Muscle spasm (PO)
- Seizure disorder (PO)
- Status epilepticus (IV)
- Seizure clusters (rectal gel)
- Seizure clusters (nasal)

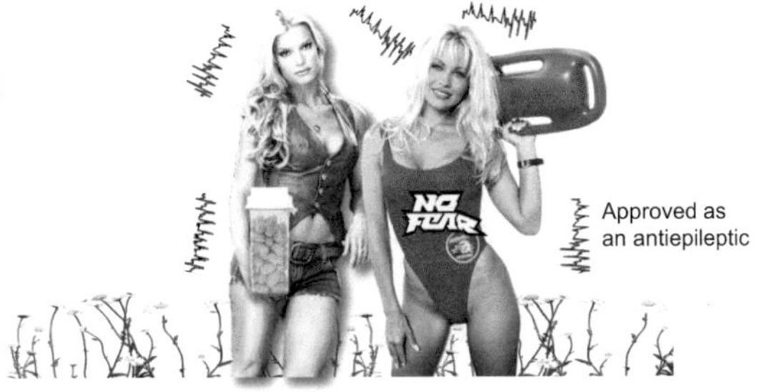

Diazepam was introduced in 1963 and was widely prescribed for "anxiety neurosis" (DSM-II). Valium is credited as the "little yellow pill" in the Rolling Stones' 1966 hit *Mother's Little Helper*, although meprobamate (Miltown) had the same reputation preceding Valium.

For anxiety, it is dosed BID to QID. Due to its rapid onset of action, diazepam is one of the more addictive benzodiazepines, but has less potential for addiction than alprazolam (Xanax).

Due to diazepam's very long half-life, abrupt discontinuation is less likely to result in withdrawal seizures compared to alprazolam. Active metabolites of diazepam include desmethyldiazepam (100-hour half-life), oxazepam (available as Serax), and temazepam (available as Restoril).

The original branded 5 mg tab

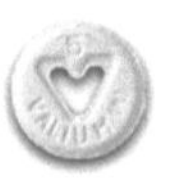

VALTOCO, approved in 2020, is an intranasal formulation of diazepam for intermittent episodes of frequent seizure activity (seizure clusters), as an alternative to diazepam rectal gel (DIASTAT). The other benzo approproved for cluster seizures is midazolam (page 64).

Diazepam is more effective for muscle spasms than other BZDs. It may be given rectally for emergency seizure control.

Diazepam is FDA-approved for alcohol withdrawal, IV or PO. An oral benzo would be used for uncomplicated withdrawal, either chlordiazepoxide (Librium) or Valium. Intravenous diazepam is the drug of choice for complicated alcohol withdrawal (delirium tremens).

Dosing: 5 mg is the standard full-strength oral dose. For anxiety, start 2 mg or 2.5 mg PO BID PRN. FDA max is 40 mg/day divided BID–QID. High doses are needed for treatment of alcohol withdrawal, e.g., 20 mg q 2 hr based on Clinical Institute Withdrawal Assessment (CIWA) score, to call physician if 5 doses given (100 mg).

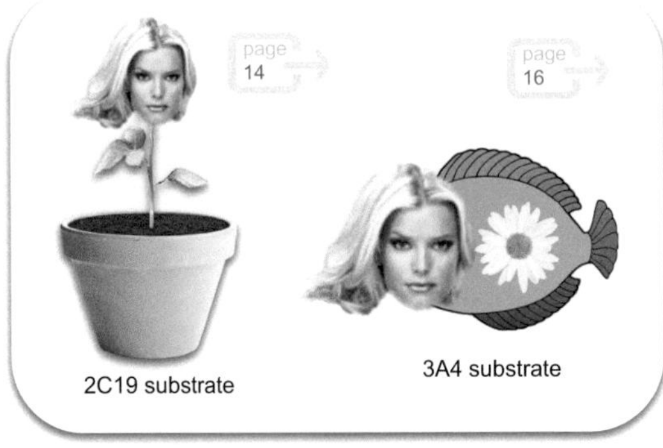

2C19 substrate

3A4 substrate

#185
1981
$1–$23

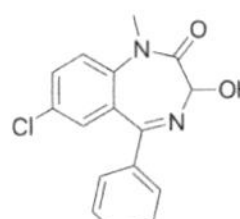

Temazepam (RESTORIL)

te MAZ e pam / REST or il

"The 'mazing Rest troll"

- Benzodiazepine
- Slow onset
- Intermediate duration
- DEA Schedule IV

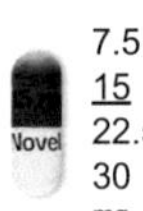

7.5
15
22.5
30
mg

FDA-approved for:

- Insomnia, short-term use

Temazepam is an intermediate duration BZD taken at bedtime for insomnia. It is never intended to be taken during the day.

Temazepam is a suitable BZD for the elderly or for those with liver disease because it metabolized by phase II conjugation as opposed to being oxidized by CYP enzymes. This applies to Lorazepam, Oxazepam and Temazepam, the "LOT" benzos.

The American Academy of Sleep Medicine (AASM) guideline (2017) states "We suggest that clinicians use temazepam as a treatment for sleep onset and sleep maintenance (vs no treatment)" based on trials of 15 mg. The direction and strength of the recommendation was "weak" and quality of the evidence was "moderate". The only other medications suggested for both onset and maintenance were the Z-drugs zolpidem (Ambien) and eszopiclone (Lunesta).

Dosing: Start 15 mg HS PRN, may increase to FDA max of 30 mg HS. Start 7.5 mg for elderly patients.

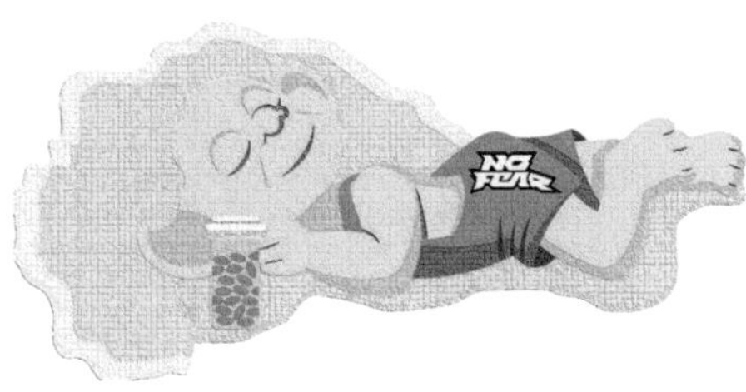

The original branded 15 mg capsule says "for sleep"

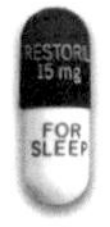

Dynamic interactions:

- Sedation
- Respiratory depression
- Do not combine with alcohol or opioids

Kinetic interactions:

- UGT2**B**15 substrate
  - Valproate (Depakote) Increases levels of "LOT" **b**enzos

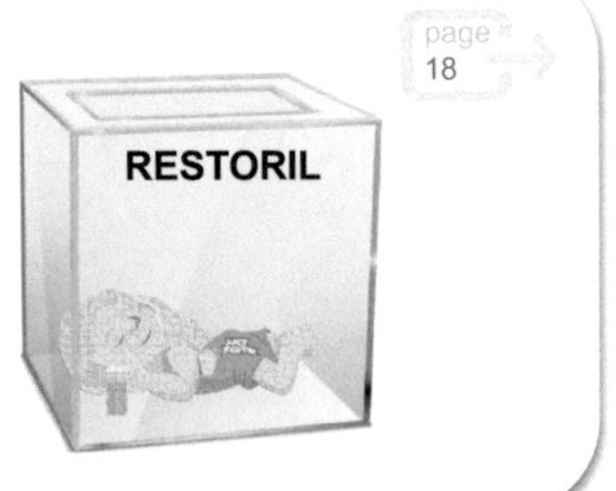

1960
$8–$14

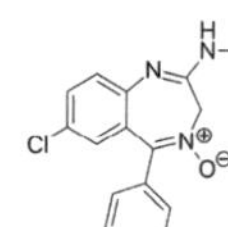

Chlordiazepoxide (LIBRIUM)

klor die as uh POK side / LIB ree um

"Lord, Liberate (me from alcohol withdrawal)"

- Benzodiazepine
- Intermediate onset
- Long duration
- DEA Schedule IV

5
10
25
mg

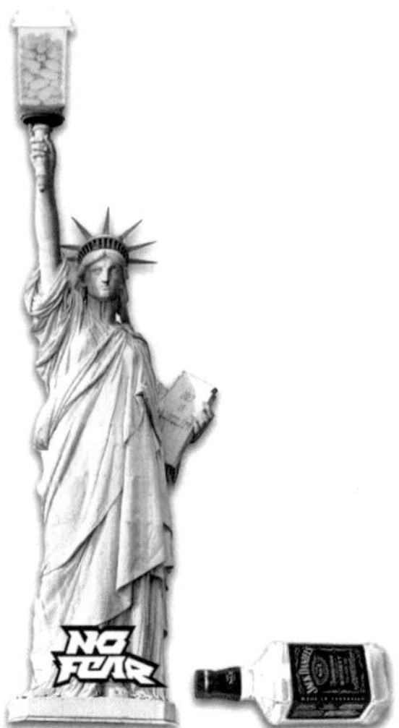

FDA-approved for:

- Anxiety (mild to moderate) 5–10 mg TID–QID
- Severe anxiety 20–25 mg TID–QID
- Preoperative anxiety 5–10 mg TID–QID
- Alcohol withdrawal 50–100 mg PRN (max 30 days)

Chlordiazepoxide (Librium) was the first benzodiazepine, available since 1960. Oral chlordiazepoxide is useful for managing uncomplicated withdrawal from alcohol or from other benzos, thanks to its long half-life. Due to Librium's tendency to accumulate, it is not very useful for any other indication. It is only available PO, so it is necessary to have IM lorazepam (Ativan) or IV diazepam (Valium) handy in the event of an alcohol-withdrawal seizure.

With regular use, chlordiazepoxide can be detected in urine a week after discontinuation. The same applies to diazepam. Contrast this to alprazolam (Xanax), which may be undetectable at 24 hours.

Dosing: See above; Taper to discontinue

Management of alcohol withdrawal

Alternatives include

- Chlordiazepoxide (Librium) - PO
- Lorazepam (Ativan) - PO, IM
- Diazepam (Valium) - PO, IV
- Midazolam (Versed) - IV
- Phenobarbital (Luminal) - PO, IV

Hospital protocols may prefer one agent over another. They are usually dosed according to a severity assessment scale such as Clinical Institute Withdrawal Assessment (CIWA). For ICU patients who are in severe withdrawal and cannot respond to questions, the Minnesota Detoxification Scale (MINDS) is used.

Consider adding haloperidol (Haldol) for a patient experiencing hallucinations or psychosis, known as delirium tremens—aka the "DT's".

Alternate mnemonic: *Cooler dies of pox (in the) Library*

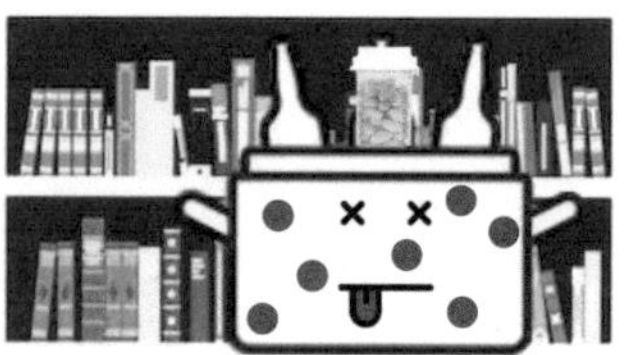

Dynamic interactions:

- Sedation
- Respiratory depression
- Do not combine with alcohol or opioids

Kinetic interactions:

- 3A4 substrate

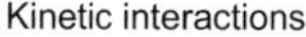

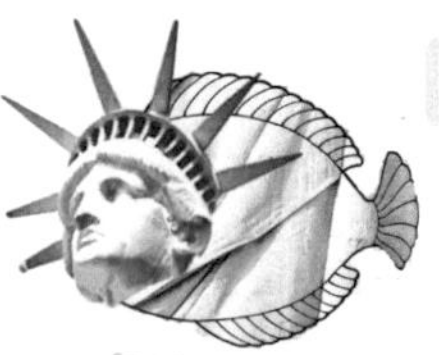

3A4 substrate

page 16

1982
$36–$102

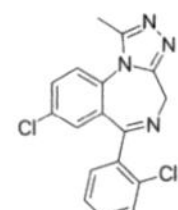

Triazolam (HALCION)

tri A zo lam / HAL see on

"HAL Tries lamenting"

- Benzodiazepine
- Intermediate onset
- Short duration
- DEA Schedule IV

0.125
0.25
mg

FDA-approved for:

- Insomnia (short term treatment)

Short tripod, short half-life of 1.5 to 5.5 hours. This is the shortest half-life of any **oral** benzodiazepine (parenteral midazolam has a half-life of 1 to 4 hours).

Triazolam was released to the US market in 1982. It became the #1 prescribed sleep medication until the early 1990s when it was found to be more dangerous than other BZDs. Risks include anterograde amnesia and sleep activities, like those seen with the Z-drugs (Ambien, etc). Triazolam has been blamed for murders and suicides.

It is now rarely prescribed by psychiatrists. However, the American Academy of Sleep Medicine (AASM) 2017 guidelines state "We suggest that clinicians use triazolam as a treatment for sleep onset insomnia (versus no treatment)". Strength of the suggestion was "weak" with "high" quality evidence and "benefits approximately equal to risks".

Due to its short half-life, triazolam is not effective for patients who experience frequent night or early morning awakening. For those with initial insomnia, the short half-life is desirable, with no morning grogginess expected.

Sublingual administration of triazolam increases bioavailability by 28% by bypassing first-pass metabolism by the liver (Scavone et al, 1986).

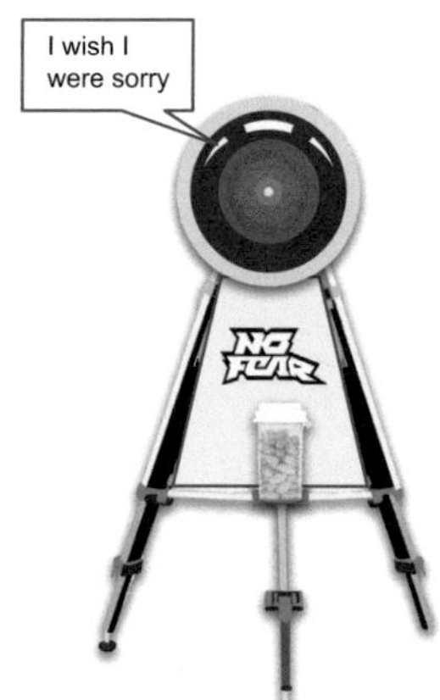

HAL 9000 from *2001: A Space Odyssey*

Dosing: Start 0.125 or 0.25 mg HS PRN. FDA max is 0.5 mg HS. Take immediately before bedtime. Use lower dose with elderly patients. Taper to discontinue.

Dynamic interactions:

- Sedation
- Respiratory depression
- Do not combine with alcohol or opioids

Kinetic interactions:

- 3A4 substrate (major)
  - Grapefruit juice, a weak 3A4 inHibitor, increases exposure to triazolam by 50%

page 16

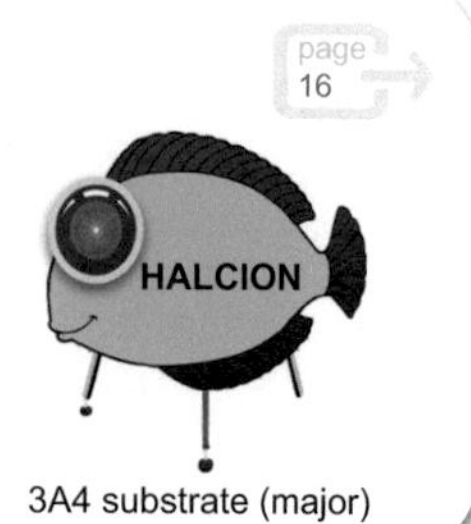

3A4 substrate (major)

1972
$62–$208

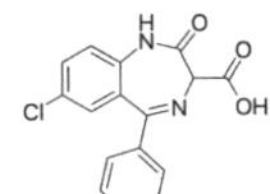

Clorazepate (TRANXENE)

klor AZ e pate / TRAN zeen

"(Cloraze)peyton Trancing"

- Benzodiazepine
- Intermediate onset
- Long duration
- DEA Schedule IV

3.75
7.5
15
mg

FDA-approved for:

- Anxiety
- Alcohol withdrawal
- Focal seizures (adjunct)

Approved as an antiepileptic

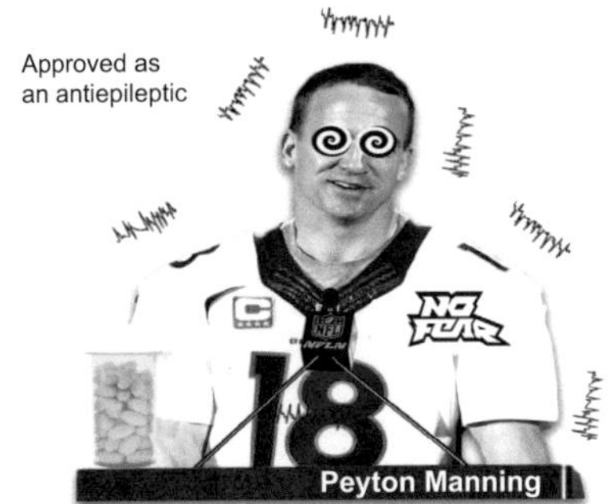

Long trance, long half-life

This benzo has a unique name, ending in -pate, rather than -pam. Clorazepate (Tranxene) is water-soluble, which is unusual among benzodiazepines. Clorazepate is a prodrug with a lipid-soluble active metabolite. Clorazepate, which cannot be absorbed from the GI tract, is hydrolyzed in the stomach to its active form, desmethyldiazepam. Desmethyldiazepam is long-lasting, and a small amount of it is further metabolised into oxazepam (Serax, shown below).

Clorazepate is rarely prescribed, so most pharmacies will not keep it in stock. The marketing slogan for Tranxene was "Awake on the job, yet anxiety controlled". It is purportedly less sedating than the average benzo. This mnemonic might have been *Transit-ing* rather than *Trance-ing* if the marketing hype was believable.

Dosing: For anxiety, start 7.5 mg QD, with target dose of 15–60 mg/day divided BID–TID; Alternatively, 15–30 mg HS; As with any antiepileptic, taper to discontinue.

Awake on the job, yet anxiety controlled
Troublesome drowsiness uncommon.
Tranxene
(CLORAZEPATE DIPOTASSIUM)

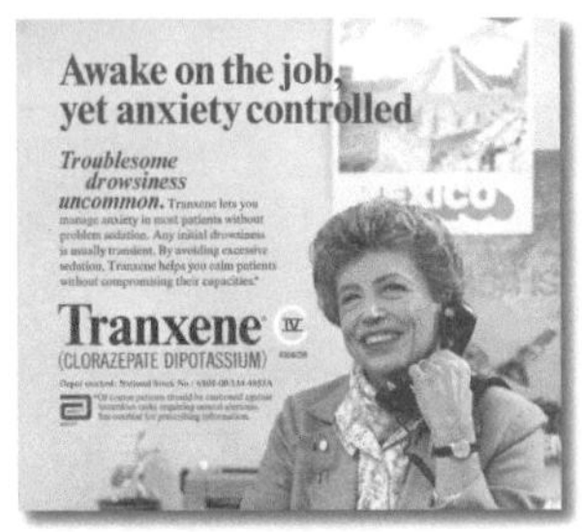

The original branded 15 mg tablet

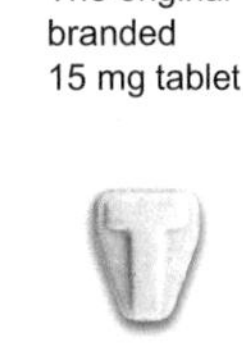

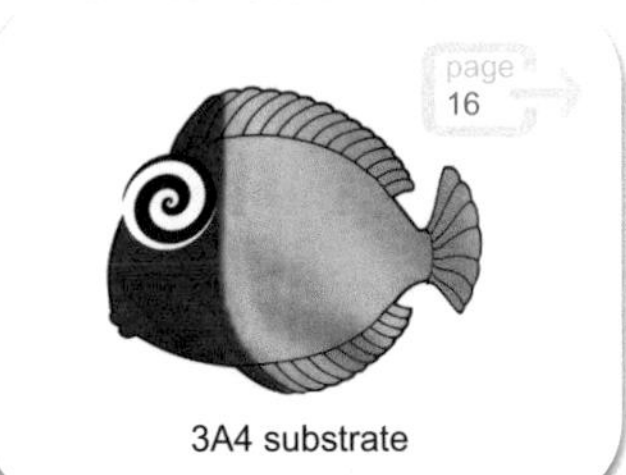

3A4 substrate

1965
$41–$126

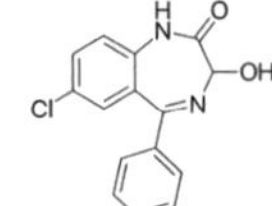

Oxazepam (SERAX)

ox A ze pam / SER ax

"Sara axed Ox"

- Benzodiazepine
- Slow onset
- Short duration
- DEA Schedule IV

10
15
30
mg

FDA-approved for:

- Anxiety
- Alcohol withdrawal (not ideal due to short half-life)

Shortened life, short half-life.

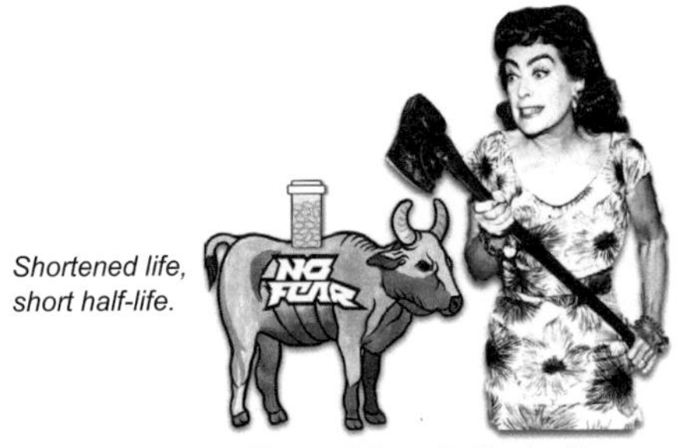

"Sera cut the ox's life short"

Among BZDs, oxazepam has the lowest fatality index and the lowest abuse potential, likely due to its slow onset of action. It is slowly absorbed and enters the brain gradually. The therapeutic effect builds over 3 hours, which is much more delayed than other BZDs (30–90 minutes). Slow onset is also the reason for the relative underutilization of oxazepam, as anxious patients may not want to wait 3 hours for relief.

Oxazepam is not involved in CYP kinetic interactions, as it is metabolized by phase II conjugation. This applies to Lorazepam, Oxazepam, and Temazepam—the "LOT" benzos. These three BZDs have no active metabolites and do not accumulate with long term use.

As expected for a rarely-prescribed old drug, oxazepam is relatively expensive, and most pharmacies do not stock it.

Dosing: The FDA approved range for anxiety is 10–30 mg TID to QID. Do not exceed 15 mg/dose for elderly patients. Taper to discontinue. Be advised smaller pharmacies will not have it in stock.

You can't set her free. But you can help her feel less anxious.
To help you relieve anxiety and tension
Serax
(oxazepam)

FREEDOM
SERAX

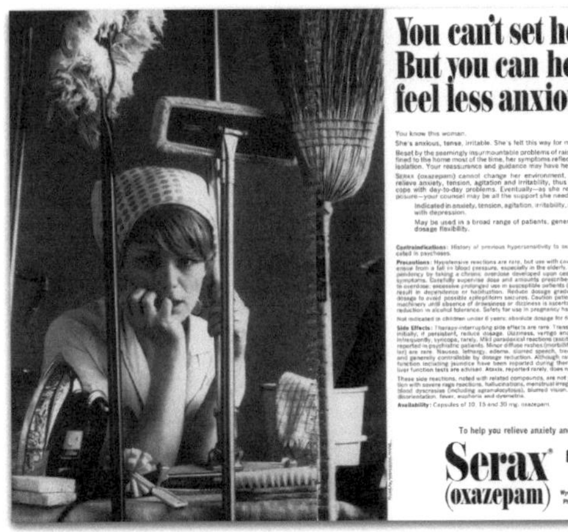

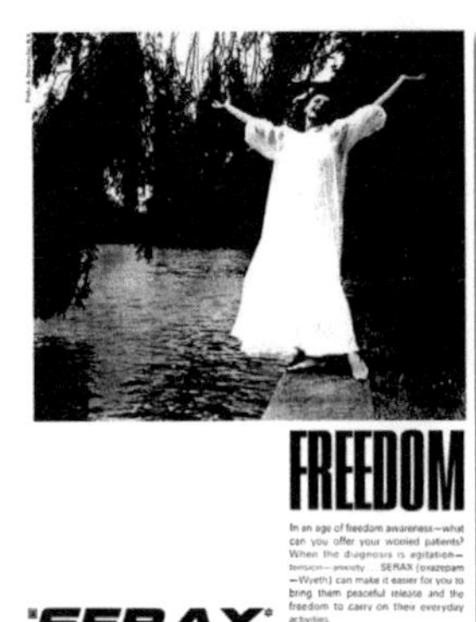

Dynamic interactions:

- Sedation
- Respiratory depression
- Do not combine with alcohol or opioids

Kinetic interactions:

- UGT2**B**15 substrate
  - Valproate (Depakote) increases blood levels of the "LOT" **b**enzos

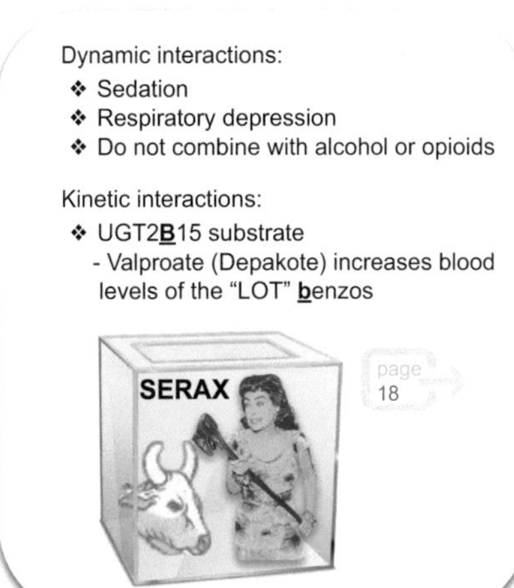

1970
$16–$31

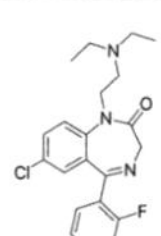

Flurazepam (DALMANE)

flure AZ e pam / DAHL mane

"Dalmatian on Floor"

- ❖ Benzodiazepine
- ❖ Intermediate onset
- ❖ Long duration
- ❖ DEA Schedule IV

15
30
mg

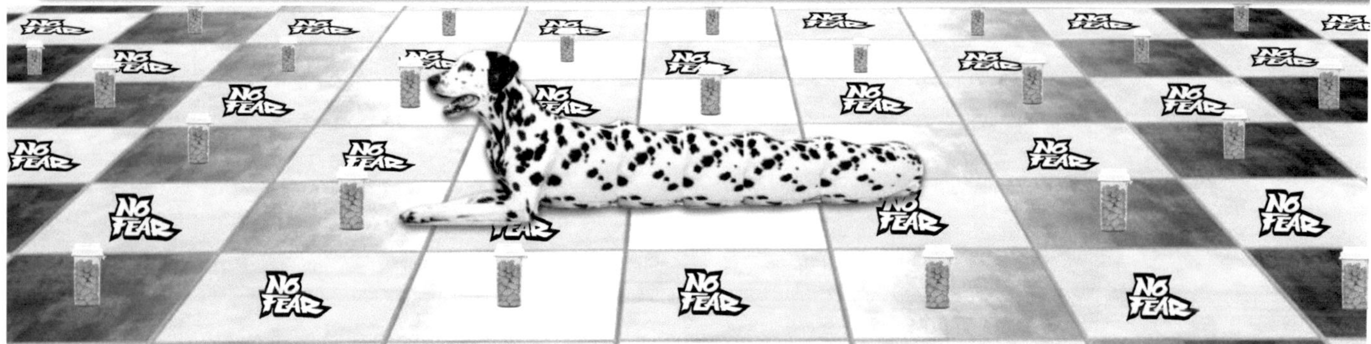

FDA-approved for
- ❖ Insomnia, short-term use

Long dog, long half-life. Flurazepam has been available in the US since 1970. We're getting into rare territory, so pharmacies are unlikely to have it in stock.

When used as a hypnotic, flurazepam's 80-hour half-life may lead to daytime grogginess and accumulation of the drug. *This dog is too long.* Prescribe temazepam (Restoril) instead.

Dosing: The FDA-approved range for insomnia is 15–30 mg HS. Do not exceed 15 mg with elderly patients. Taper to discontinue.

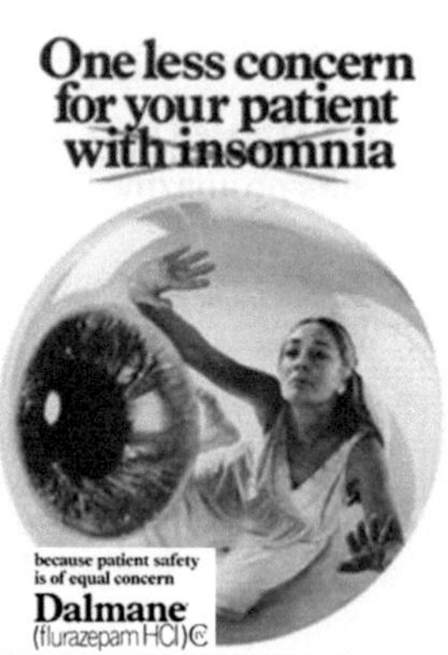

Dynamic interactions:
- ❖ Sedation
- ❖ Respiratory depression
- ❖ Do not combine with alcohol or opioids

page 16

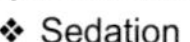
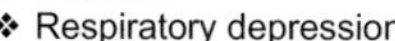

Kinetic interactions:
- ❖ 3A4 substrate

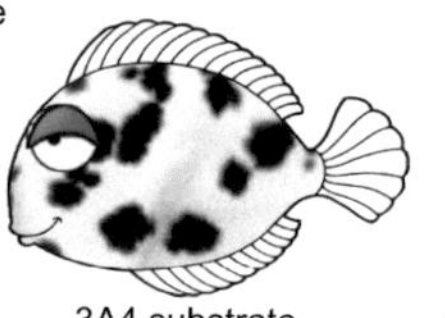

3A4 substrate

1979
$19–$56

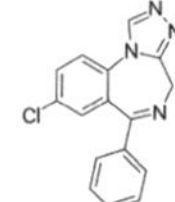

Estazolam (PROSOM)

es TAE zo lam / PRO som

"Stay Prostrate & som(nolent)"

- ❖ Benzodiazepine
- ❖ Intermediate onset
- ❖ Intermediate duration
- ❖ DEA Schedule IV

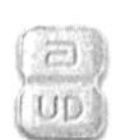

1
2
mg

FDA-approved for:
- ❖ Insomnia, short-term use

Estazolam is a rarely prescribed benzodiazepine not stocked by many pharmacies. As the trade name suggests, Prosom was marketed for insomnia. Its intermediate half-life is well suited for this indication.

Dosing: Start: 1 mg HS PRN. Max dose is 2 mg. For elderly patients, start 0.5 mg HS. Taper to discontinue.

I'm hoping this guy stays prostrate for an intermediate length of time.

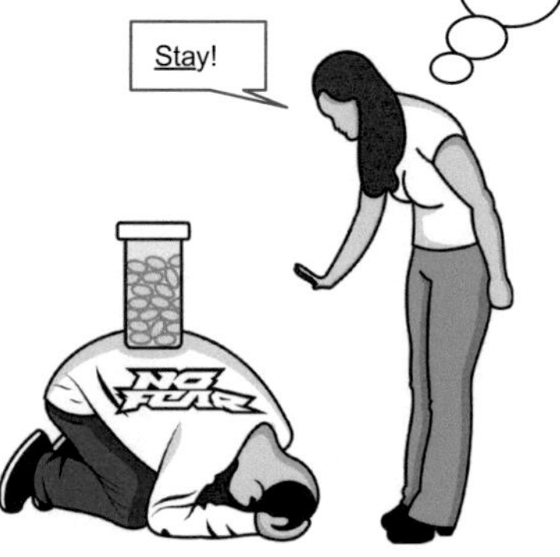

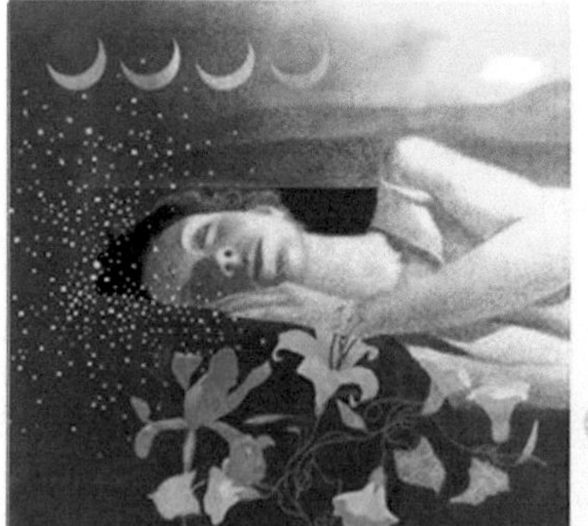

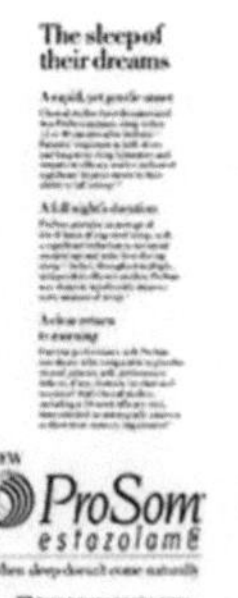

3A4 substrate

page 16

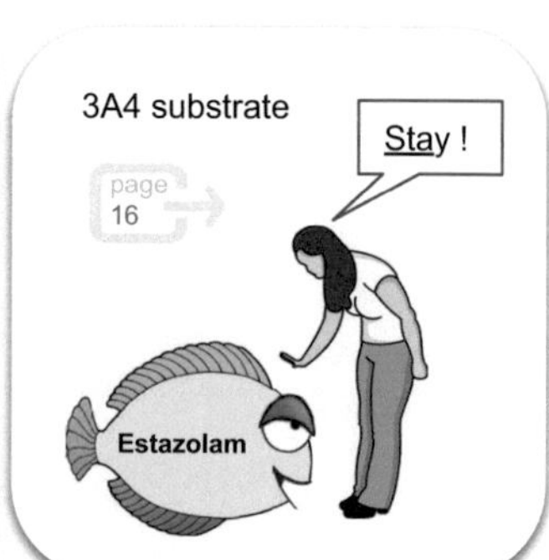

1977
$701–$746

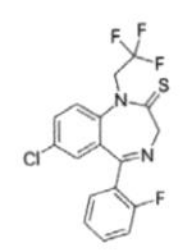

Quazepam (DORAL)

qua ze pam / DOR al

"Quasimodo & Dora"

- ❖ Benzodiazepine
- ❖ Intermediate onset
- ❖ Long duration
- ❖ DEA Schedule IV

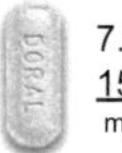

7.5
15
mg

FDA-approved for:

- ❖ Insomnia, short-term use

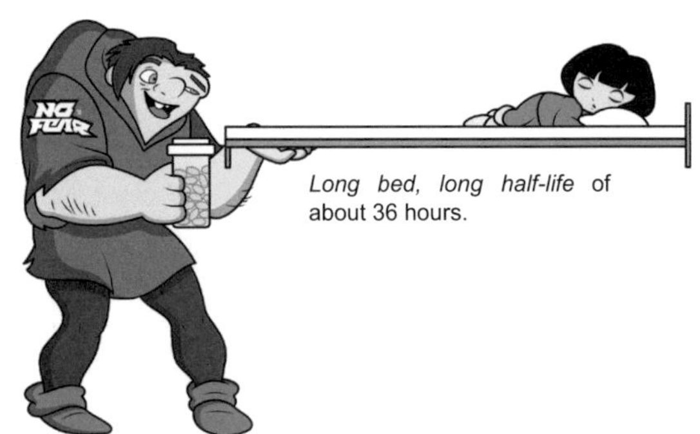

Long bed, long half-life of about 36 hours.

Structurally, quazepam is a benzodiazepine, but its mechanism is closer to a nonbenzodiazepine Z-drug such as zolpidem (Ambien). You might say its a "quasi-Z-drug". Compared to other benzos, quazepam has less potential to induce tolerance or respiratory depression.

Quazepam has a longer duration of action than Z-drugs, which may be longer than desired for a night's sleep. There may be marked next day impairment due to accumulation of quazepam and its long-acting metabolites. It is not recommended.

Of the older benzodiazepines, quazepam is the most expensive and the least prescribed. Health insurance plans won't cover it and the pharmacy would have to special-order it.

Doral is better known as a brand of cigarettes that debuted in 1969, preceding the pharmaceutical (1977).

Dosing: The FDA-approved dose range is 7.5–15 mg HS.

Dynamic interactions:

- ❖ Sedation
- ❖ Respiratory depression
- ❖ Do not combine with alcohol or opioids

page 16

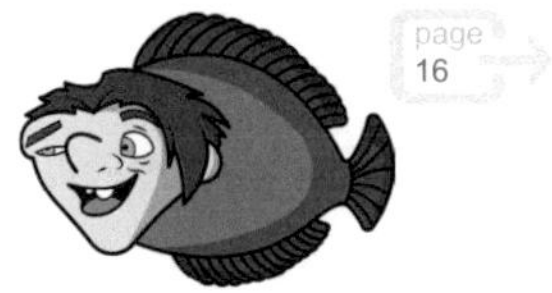

Kinetic interactions:

- ❖ 3A4 substrate

3A4 substrate

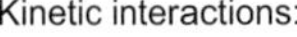

2011
$36–$904

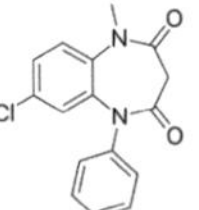

Clobazam (Onfi)

KLOE ba zam / ON fee

"Clobber On wi-fi"

- ❖ 1,5 benzodiazepine
- ❖ Rapid onset
- ❖ Long duration
- ❖ DEA Schedule IV

10
20
mg

FDA-approved for:

- ❖ Seizures of Lennox-Gastaut syndrome (LGS)

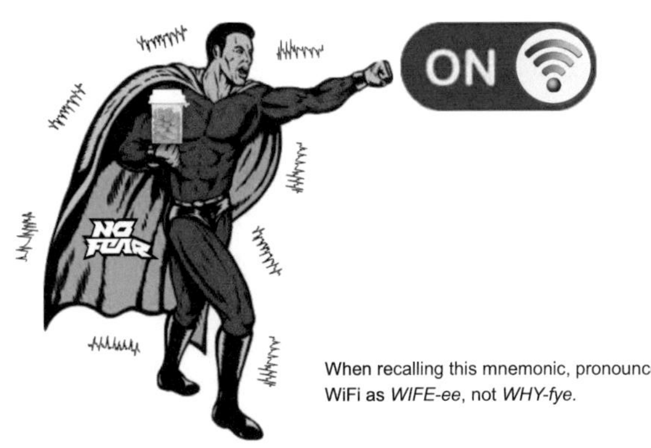

When recalling this mnemonic, pronounce WiFi as *WIFE-ee*, not *WHY-fye*.

Clobazam, long available in other countries, was finally FDA-approved in the US in 2011 for adjunctive treatment of seizures associated with Lennox-Gastaut Syndrome (ages 2 years or older). Outside of the US it was marketed as an anxiolytic since 1975 and an anticonvulsant since 1984.

Lennox-Gastaut syndrome (LGS), pronounced *gas-TOE*, is a type of childhood-onset epilepsy characterized by the triad of multiple seizure types, intellectual impairment, and characteristic EEG findings.

Clobazam is a Schedule IV controlled substance like all of the other benzos. While most benzos are 3A4 substrates, clobazam is a 2C19 substrate. Cannabidiol (CBD oil), also approved for Lennox-Gastaut syndrome, is a 2C19 inHibitor that increases exposure to clobazam 3-fold. Ingestion of alcohol increases the blood concentration of clobazam by about 50%.

So, what is so special about clobazam? Probably not much. It does have a unique structure. Clobazam is the only available 1,5 BZD. Unlike the 1,4 BZDs, clobazam is thought to be advantageous due to a rapid onset of action, broad spectrum of activity, and long half-life. However, the other benzos were not directly compared to clobazam for treatment of LGS.

The clinical advantage of clobazam is it appears to be less sedating than other benzos.

Dosing: For those >30 kg start 5 mg BID x 1 week, then 10 mg BID x 1 week, then to target dose of 20 mg BID. Maximum is 40 mg/day. Use a half-strength dose for 2C19 poor metabolizers. Also, as with any antiepileptic, taper to discontinue.

Dynamic interactions:

page 14

- ❖ Sedation
- ❖ Respiratory depression
- ❖ Do not combine with alcohol or opioids

Kinetic interactions:

- ❖ While most benzos are 3A4 substrates, clobazam is a 2C19 substrate (major)
- ❖ Cannabidiol (CBD), also approved for Lennox-Gastaut syndrome, is a 2C19 inHibitor that increases exposure to clobazam 3-fold.

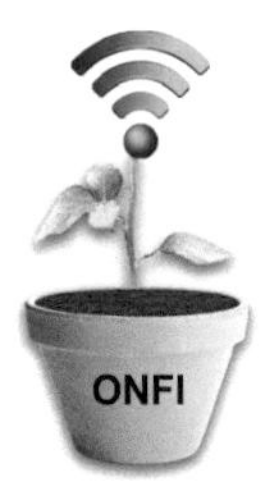

2C19 substrate (major)

1975
$15

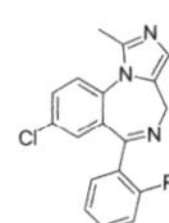

Midazolam (VERSED)

mye DAZ oh lam / ver SED

"Midas' Versus..."

- ❖ Parenteral benzodiazepine
- ❖ DEA Schedule IV

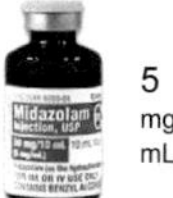

5 mg/mL

FDA-approved for:

- ❖ Procedural sedation
- ❖ Preoperative sedation (IM, PO syrup)
- ❖ General anesthesia induction and maintenance
- ❖ Mechanical ventilation sedation
- ❖ Seizure clusters (nasal spray)

Midazolam (Versed) is a benzodiazepine primarily administered intravenously. It is not used in psychiatry. Midazolam has the shortest half-life of any benzodiazepine, of 1 to 4 hours.

Midazolam is not available as a pill, but a cherry syrup is available for preoperative sedation, for instance in dentist offices. Prior to availability of the syrup, some doctors mixed the parenteral midazolam solution into acetaminophen syrup for pediatric preoperative sedation (Shrestha et al, 2007).

A few US states use midazolam to induce sleep for death penalty executions, in combination with pancuronium bromide (to paralyze the diaphragm), and potassium chloride (to stop the heart).

Midazolam is one of the few water-soluble BZDs. Its unique chemical structure makes it water soluble at pH < 4, and lipid-soluble at physiologic pH so that it can cross the blood-brain barrier. Water soluble medications are less painful upon injection.

Water-solubility makes midazolam the only BZD that can be administered intranasally. It is given by paramedics when transporting highly agitated patients. The injectable liquid can be put in a mucosal atomization device and used for acute seizure management, as an alternative to diazepam rectal solution (De Haan et al, 2010). If the nasal spray is used, first give lidocaine nasal spray because the low-pH midazolam spray is going to sting. The nasal spray formulation (NAYZILAM) was finally FDA-approved in 2019 for cluster seizures.

As a side note, you won't see drug users crushing and snorting BZD pills (e.g., Xanax) because they are not water soluble and therefore cannot be absorbed through the nasal mucosa.

Alternate mnemonic: *"the Verse said by Midas".*

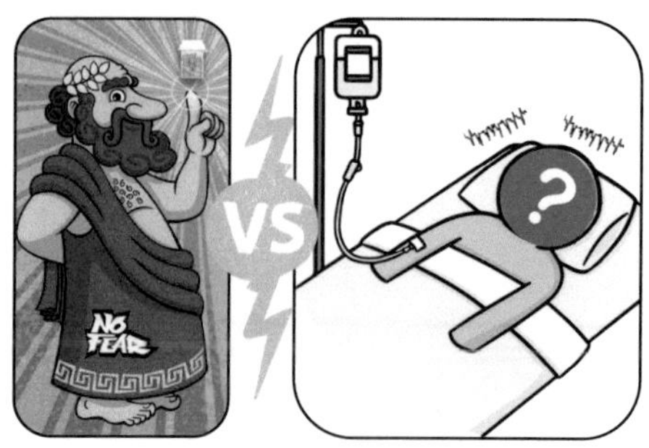

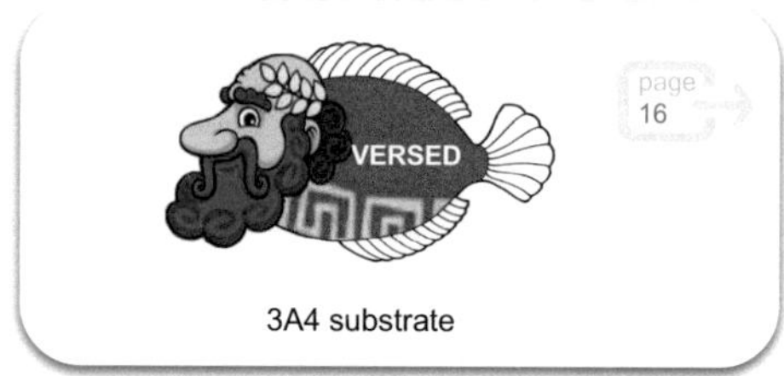

page 16

3A4 substrate

1987
$61

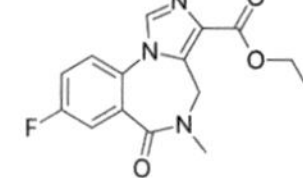

Flumazenil (ROMAZICON)

floo MAZ e nil / ro MAZ e con

"Flume a 'zepine"

- ❖ GABA(A) receptor antagonist
- ❖ Antidote for BZD overdose

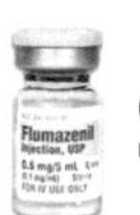

0.1 mg/mL

FDA-approved for:

- ❖ Benzodiazepine overdose
- ❖ Benzodiazepine sedation reversal

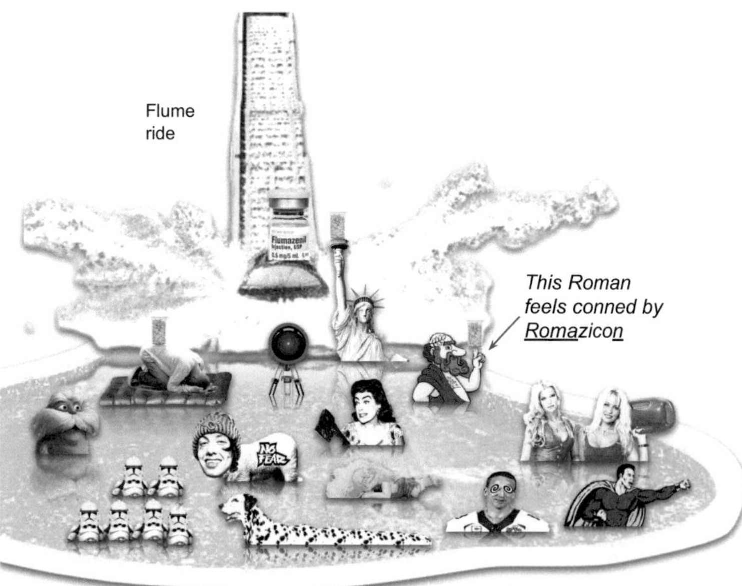

Dosing: 0.2 mg IV x 1, wait 30 seconds and give 0.3 mg IV x 1 PRN, then wait 30 seconds and give 0.5 mg IV PRN up to six doses for maximum of 5 mg total; If re-sedation occurs, repeat 0.5 mg IV (2 doses 30 seconds apart) q 20 minutes for a maximum of 3 mg/hour.

Flumazenil, the antidote for BZD overdose, is an antagonist at the BZD binding site on the GABA(A) receptor complex. Flumazenil also blocks nonbenzodiazepine Z-drugs. It does not block barbiturates. It is available for IV and intranasal delivery. Duration of action is only 30–60 minutes, necessitating multiple doses.

Since the body does not produce endogenous BZDs, flumazenil has no effect when administered in the absence of a BZD.

Flumazenil has a **black box warning** to prepare for the possibility of the patient having a seizure. If the person is physically dependent on BZDs, seizure is highly likely. Flumazenil is unlikely to cause a seizure for a person who overdosed on a bottle of someone else's benzo.

The usual consequences of a large BZD overdose are profound sedation and possible coma. A standalone BZD overdose does not typically cause respiratory arrest but can be life threatening due to aspiration.

Due to risk of seizure, flumazenil nasal spray is not dispensed to family members for home use (as is done with naloxone for opioids).

Another medication that blocks benzodiazepine binding in the brain is physostigmine, a cholinesterase inhibitor that is more commonly used to reverse anticholinergic toxicity.

About the author:

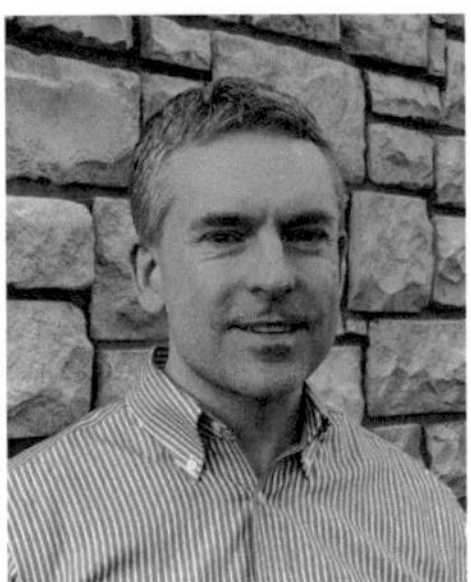

Dr Jason Cafer is Medical Director for Behavioral Health Services at SSM Health/St. Mary's Hospital in Jefferson City, Missouri where he serves as attending physician for a bustling 20-bed acute inpatient psychiatric ward. He graduated from University of Missouri-Columbia School of Medicine in 2003 and completed Psychiatric Residency at the same institution in 2007. He is a diplomate of the American Board of Psychiatry and Neurology and is also board-certified in Addiction Medicine by the American Board of Preventive Medicine. Prior to St. Mary's, he practiced inpatient psychiatry at Fulton State Hospital and outpatient at Comprehensive Health Systems. In 2007 he founded Iconic Health, a medical informatics startup that obtained angel round funding. He was Principal Investigator for Phase I and II Small Business Innovation Research (SBIR) grants for "Online Rural Telepsychiatry Platform" (2007-2009) funded by the United States Department of Agriculture. He is the inventor of United States Patent US8255241B2 which was the subject of an SBIR grant awarded by the Department of Health and Human Services for "Medication IconoGraphs: Visualization of Complex Medication Regimens". He completed *Cafers' Psychopharmacology* while serving as preceptor for Stephens College Master of Physician Assistant Studies program. Dr. Cafer aspires to provide an online Continuing Medical Education course for psychiatrists and other medical professionals.

Also available:

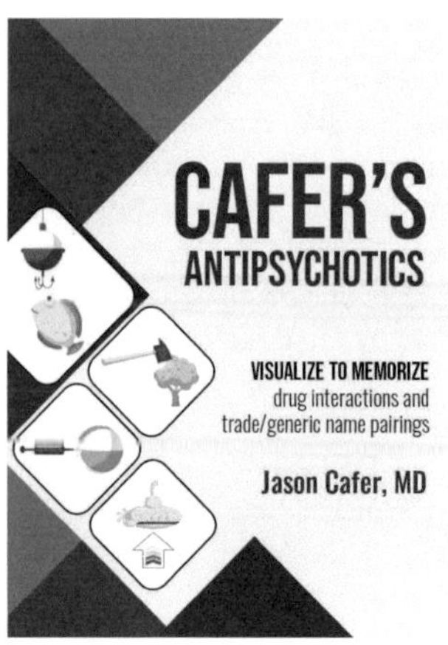

Cafer's Antipsychotics
39 medications

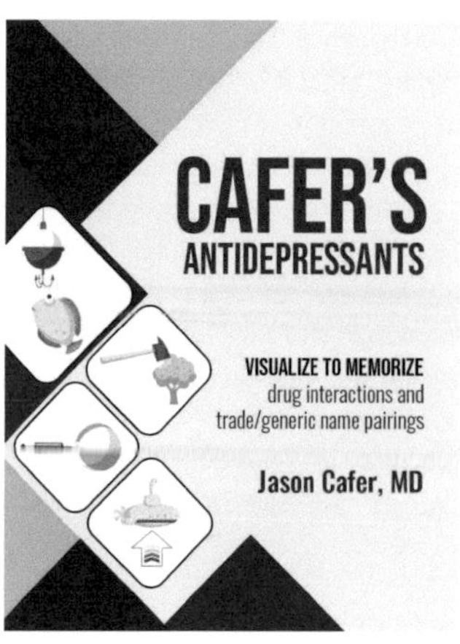

Cafer's Antidepressants
36 medications

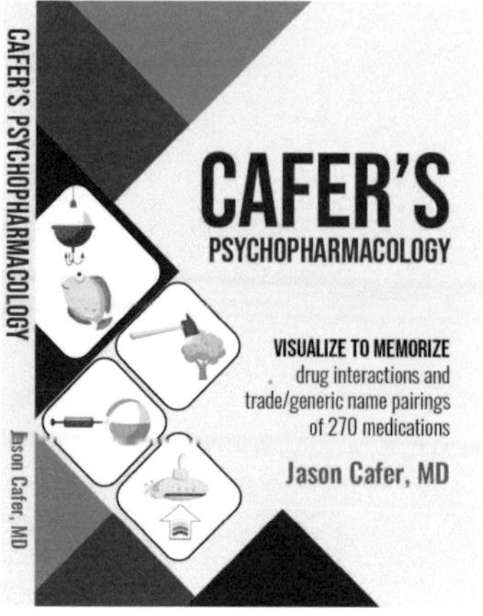

Cafer's Psychopharmacology
270 medications

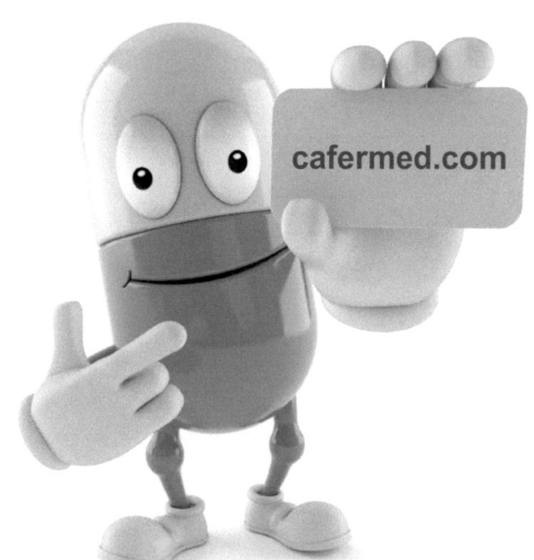

Visit cafermed.com and use promo code **EMBIGGEN** for a discount on the big book, Cafer's Psychopharmacology: Visualize to Memorize 270 Medication Mascots.

Made in United States
Troutdale, OR
09/29/2023